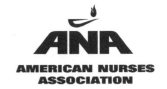

Care Coordination: The Game Changer

How Nursing is Revolutionizing Quality Care

Gerri Lamb, PhD, RN, FAAN – Editor

American Nurses Association
Silver Spring, Maryland
2014

D1361673

The American Nurses Association (ANA) is a national professional association. This ANA publication— *Care Coordination: The Game Changer - How Nursing is Revolutionizing Quality Care*—reflects the thinking of the nursing profession on various issues and should be reviewed in conjunction with state board of nursing policies and practices. State law, rules, and regulations govern the practice of nursing, while — *Care Coordination: The Game Changer – How Nursing is Revolutionizing Quality Care* guides nurses in the application of their professional skills and responsibilities.

American Nurses Association

8515 Georgia Avenue, Suite 400

Silver Spring, MD 20910-3492

1-800-274-4ANA

www.NursingWorld.org

Published by the Nursing Knowledge Center

www.nursingknowledgecenter.org

ISBN: 978-1-55810-543-0   SAN: 851-3481   08/2018R

First printing: December 2014. Second printing: November 2015. Fourth printing: August 2017. Fifth printing: January 2018. Sixth Printing: August 2018.

For my mother, Dorothy Saffron Lamb
My greatest cheerleader and the inspiration for this book

Contents

Section 2.   *Care Coordination: Practice and Leadership*

Section 3. *Improving Quality Through Effective Care Coordination*

Section 4. *Transforming Healthcare Practice and Policy*

Contributors

VOLUME EDITOR AND CHAPTER AUTHOR

Gerri Lamb, PhD, RN, FAAN
Associate Professor, Arizona State University, College of Nursing and Health Innovation, Herberger Institute for Design and the Arts, Phoenix, Arizona

CHAPTER AUTHORS

Corrine Abraham, DNP, RN
Nurse Fellow, VA Quality Scholars Program, Atlanta VA Medical Center; Clinical Assistant Professor, Nell Hodgson Woodruff School of Nursing, Emory University, Atlanta, Georgia

Richard C. Antonelli, MD, MS
Medical Director of Integrated Care and of Physician Relations and Outreach, Boston Children's Hospital; Faculty, Harvard Medical School, Boston, Massachusetts

Gail E. Armstrong, DNP, PhD(c), ACNS-BC, CNE
Associate Professor, University of Colorado College of Nursing, Aurora, Colorado

Patricia S. Button, EdD, RN
Managing Director, Clinical Architecture, The Advisory Board Company, Washington, D.C.

Karen Jiggins Colorafi, MBA, RN, CPEHR, CPHIT
EHR Nurse Consultant, Healthcare Practice Services, Ltd., Phoenix, Arizona

Ingrid M. Hopkins Duva, PhD RN
Nurse Fellow, National VA Quality Scholars Program, Atlanta, Georgia

Patricia Dykes, PhD, RN, FAAN, FACMI

Senior Nurse Scientist; Program Director, Center for Patient Safety Research and Practice; Program Director, Center for Nursing Excellence, Brigham and Women's Hospital; Assistant Professor,Harvard Medical School, Boston, Massachusetts

Sheila Haas, PhD, RN, FAAN

Professor, Marcella Niehoff School of Nursing, Loyola University, Chicago, Illinois

Rosemary Kennedy, PhD, RN, MBA, FAAN

Associate Professor, Associate Dean of Strategic Initiatives, Thomas Jefferson University, Jefferson School of Nursing, Philadelphia, Pennsylvania

Laura K. Heermann Langford, PhD, RN

Director, Nursing Informatics, HWCIR, Intermountain Healthcare; Assistant Professor (Clinical), College of Nursing, University of Utah, Salt Lake City, Utah

Steven J. Miller, MA

Business Manager, Sinclair Home Care Aging in Place, University of Missouri, Columbia, Missouri

Katy Musterman, MBA, RN

Manager of Nursing Services Aging In Place, TigerPlace Care Coordinator, University of Missouri, Columbia, Missouri

Lori L. Popejoy, PhD, RN

Associate Professor, University of Missouri, Columbia, Missouri

Marilyn Rantz, PhD, RN, FAAN

Curators' Professor, MU Sinclair School of Nursing; Helen E. Nahm Chair, MU Sinclair School of Nursing; University Hospitals and Clinics Professor of Nursing; Executive Director, Aging In Place and TigerPlace; Associate Director, MU Interdisciplinary Center on Aging, University of Missouri, Columbia, Missouri

Gina Rogers

Consultant and Founding Executive Director, Massachusetts Child Health Quality Coalition (CHQC), Watertown, Massachusetts

Lipika Samal, MD, MPH
Instructor of Medicine, Harvard Medical School; Associate Physician, Division of General Medicine and Primary Care, Brigham and Women's Hospital, Boston, Massachusetts

Madeline H. Schmitt, PhD, RN, FAAN
Professor Emerita, University of Rochester School of Nursing, Rochester, New York

Cheryl Schraeder, PhD, RN, FAAN
Associate Professor and Director of Policy and Practice Initiatives, Institute for Healthcare Innovation, University of Illinois College of Nursing, Chicago, Illinois

Daryl Sharp, PhD, PMHCNS-BC, NPP
Associate Dean for Faculty Development and Diversity, University of Rochester School of Nursing, Rochester, New York

Paul Shelton, EdD
Senior Research Specialist, Institute for Healthcare Innovation, University of Illinois College of Nursing, Chicago, Illinois

Nan M. Solomons, MS
Data Analyst, MaineHealth Center for Quality and Safety, Portland, Maine; Doctoral student, Arizona State University College of Nursing and Health Innovation, Phoenix, Arizona

Beth Ann Swan, PhD, CRNP, FAAN
Dean and Professor, Jefferson School of Nursing, Thomas Jefferson University, Philadelphia, Pennsylvania

Donna Zazworsky, MS, RN, CCM, FAAN
Vice President, Community Health and Continuum Care, Carondelet Health Network, Tucson, Arizona

About the American Nurses Association

The American Nurses Association (ANA) is the only full-service professional organization representing the interests of the nation's 3.1 million registered nurses through its constituent/state nurses associations and its organizational affiliates. The ANA advances the nursing profession by fostering high standards of nursing practice, promoting the rights of nurses in the workplace, projecting a positive and realistic view of nursing, and by lobbying the Congress and regulatory agencies on health care issues affecting nurses and the public.

About Nursesbooks.org, the Publishing Program of ANA

Nursesbooks.org publishes books on ANA core issues and programs, including ethics, leadership, quality, specialty practice, advanced practice, and the profession's enduring legacy. Best known for the foundational documents of the profession on nursing ethics, scope and standards of practice, and social policy, Nursesbooks.org is the publisher for the professional, career-oriented nurse, reaching and serving nurse educators, administrators, managers, and researchers as well as staff nurses in the course of their professional development.

Introduction

My path to understanding the value of care coordination has been a long one, full of many serendipitous opportunities, as well as ones I doggedly pursued intent on playing a role in shaping its future in nursing and health care. I have had the great fortune to work with and learn from leaders and visionaries in the field and to serve on numerous committees and workgroups aimed at improving care coordination practice, education, and research. After several decades of leading projects, conducting and consulting on studies, and thinking deeply about care coordination, I considered myself fairly knowledgeable, even occasionally expert, in some areas. I was not prepared for the most powerful lesson of my career, a personal one.

My experience of caring for my mother in the last months of her life emblazoned the importance of care coordination on my heart and in my mind. It drives my passion for this work and my beliefs about what all nurses and health professionals must understand about the power and centrality of care coordination in health care. I start this book with my mother's and my story to explain why I believe care coordination is *the* game changer for improving healthcare quality and safety.

My mother, Dorothy Saffron Lamb, was a vibrant and confident woman. At 85, she insisted on using her maiden name in all of her correspondence and told me that if I didn't include it in her obituary she would come back to haunt me. Our favorite family stories center around her risk-taking adventures. She was the one who took my young son canoeing for the first time. Fortunately, I didn't know for some time that she chose to do this in a swamp in Florida surrounded by alligators. This was pretty typical for her.

My mother lived for a number of years with several chronic diagnoses, including leukemia and heart failure. She took her illnesses in stride, took her prescribed medications (most of the time), and remained very active. Like many other individuals her age with whom I have worked as a nurse, she was selective about what she chose to understand and do about her chronic conditions. I used to tease her that her professed ignorance about heart failure was a great embarrassment to me as a nurse. I knew she knew what she was about—and she knew that I knew that she was purposely ignoring information that was an obstacle to her staying positive and active.

And then everything changed. My mother started having pain and shortness of breath and a variety of other symptoms. Her primary care physician followed her lead and focused on non-invasive treatments and palliative care. My mother turned to me to help her interpret her symptoms, to intervene with a growing list of physicians and specialists, and to advocate for her needs and preferences—all of the things we currently consider patient-centered care coordination. As my mother's health and ability to care for herself deteriorated, I spent more and more time talking with her friends and neighbors who were concerned about her and with the professionals caring for her.

One particular event stands out for me as the sentinel moment when I realized that all of my experience in developing and leading care coordination and case management programs, and in conducting research in this area, made little difference in making the system work for my mother. She called me from her physician's office saying he wanted to hospitalize her. She was convinced that if she went into the hospital she would not come out. So, as daughter and expert care coordinator, I sprang into action from 2,000 miles away. I convinced her doctor to initiate home care and oxygen treatment. And then waited and waited. The physician's office closed. There was no follow-up, home care was not initiated, and no oxygen was delivered. And thus, I became just like every other family member who tries to make the system work for their loved ones—adrift, frustrated, and frightened.

Care coordination, as you will read over and over in this book, is the glue that makes the healthcare system a safe and coherent place. Without it, people we care about, people we serve as nurses and other health professionals have great difficulty navigating from provider to provider, from setting to setting. It truly is possible to get "lost in the system." In spite of all my experience, in spite of all my best efforts, my mother and I got lost over and over again in systems that were not connected and between providers who did not communicate with each other. Connections, communication, integration, patient-centeredness, these are the elements of care coordination that are so vital to the patient experience and to achieving our national goals for quality and safety.

This book, *Care Coordination: The Game Changer*, focuses on the power of care coordination to transform health care. In these pages, care coordination is situated within the current context of healthcare reform and the national agenda for improving health care in the United States. We highlight the role of nurses in making care coordination the centerpiece of a safe, effective, patient-centered, timely, efficient, and equitable healthcare system—the vision set forward by the Institute of Medicine in *Crossing the Quality Chasm* over a decade ago and still to be realized. Certainly, nursing is not alone in this effort. Many other professions, including social work and medicine, stand side-by-side with nurses as champions for care coordination as they have for decades. The nursing profession has a unique opportunity to advance healthcare reform through its expertise in care coordination.

This book weaves the story of care coordination and nursing within the major themes of health care today. Together, the chapters cover the spectrum from the current context of health reform and the national quality agenda to the expected outcomes of care coordination and opportunities for educational and policy reform. Care coordination is the lens we use to examine nursing's contributions to national quality and safety goals. As you will see, it offers a powerful example of how core nursing practices, such as care coordination, transform and revolutionize health care.

Chapter 1 sets the stage for everything that follows. Within its pages, care coordination is defined and tied closely to the goals for improving the quality of health care in the United States. The current popularity of care coordination is explored in the context of the significant changes transpiring in our healthcare system. Nursing's significant role in the development of many care coordination models is highlighted. Recognizing nursing's impact on care coordination's past is critical to fully understanding how powerful nurses are and will be in the emerging story of new care coordination models and practices.

The chapters in Section 1 provide the foundation for understanding why care coordination is in the national spotlight and why it is likely to stay there for some time to come. In Chapter 2, Armstrong lays out the quality agenda in the United States and describes the plethora of national initiatives designed to improve quality and safety, including those that have been initiated within the nursing community. Abraham provides a rich set of frameworks and tools for understanding and improving quality and safety in Chapter 3.

Section 2 begins the deep dive into care coordination. In Chapter 4, Schraeder and Shelton conduct a thorough review of care coordination models, detailing elements associated with their effectiveness. They highlight the roles that nurses have played in the evolution and implementation of these models. In Chapter 5, Lamb, Schmitt, and Sharp describe how nurses can recognize and improve care coordination in their practice. They identify ways that nurses are being prepared to take on new care coordination roles in evolving delivery models, including patient-centered medical homes. Chapter 6 addresses the important role of nursing leaders in advancing care coordination. Duva proposes numerous strategies that nurses in both informal and formal leadership roles can use to heighten the visibility and impact of care coordination interventions.

Section 3 focuses on what we know about the relationship between care coordination interventions and important quality and safety outcomes, as well as the emerging role of health information technology in supporting care coordination. In Chapter 7,

Colorafi, Solomons, and Lamb examine research linking care coordination with hospital admission and readmission rates. Haas and Swan propose the use of a dynamic logic model to capture the impact of care coordination on patient and family outcomes in Chapter 8. In Chapter 9, Kennedy, Button, Dykes, Langford, and Samal detail the current state of health information technology in care coordination practice and help us to anticipate future developments.

The final section of the book provides real-life examples of nurses and interprofessional teams who have led the development of innovative care coordination practice models and are in the process of translating them for national healthcare policy. In Chapter 10, Antonelli and Rogers advance a new collaborative model for care coordination. They highlight the significant role that family members play in care coordination. The amount of time families spend in coordinating care is awe-inspiring. In Chapter 11, Zazworsky describes how nurses in one organization capitalized on their extensive experience to lead a project funded by the Center for Medicare and Medicaid Services to reduce preventable hospital readmissions. And finally, in Chapter 12, Rantz, Popejoy, Musterman, and Miller tell the inspiring story of Tiger Place, the realization of their vision of what care coordination can accomplish for improving quality of care and life for older adults.

The contributions to this book tell a powerful story of care coordination's past, present, and future. It is a story that is rich in themes and goals that will resonate for all nurses and other health professionals. It has taken many years for care coordination to be understood and recognized as central to health care quality for all Americans. It is only recently that the dots between care coordination and patient-centered care and teamwork have been connected—essential insights that are threaded through the history, science, and practice of nurses and the nursing profession. Most of the care coordination practices and models you will read about in this book are deeply rooted in nursing and reflect nursing's values and commitments to making health care work for patients and families. Nursing has had a very significant hand in shaping the care coordination models that are so evident today.

The story of care coordination is still very much in play and unfolding in the current dialogue about improving health and health care. Nursing's imprint on emerging models and care coordination policies are evident. The chapters of this book stand on the shoulders of many nurses and other professionals who believed deeply in the value of care coordination and created a strong foundation for its becoming the cornerstone of a patient-centered, high-quality, healthcare system.

We are at a pivotal moment in the history of care coordination. As you will see throughout this book, it is not coincidental that the power of care coordination for integrating and personalizing a fragmented and impersonal healthcare system has been recognized. Nurses have been a vital force in preparing for this time, in developing and testing new care coordination models, and in building the cache of expertise and experience essential for care coordination to achieve its intended goals in transforming health care. Nurses in every practice setting are revolutionizing quality care through expert care coordination. The message of this book, and one we hope you will find meaningful and will inspire you to action, is about opportunity and urgency. There is still much work ahead to fully realize the promise of care coordination for improving the health of our nation. Realizing this promise has been an enduring commitment and passion for the nursing profession—and in great evidence in all you will read here. Our patients and our family members like my mother rely on and need effective care coordination—it is the hallmark of an effective and caring healthcare system.

Gerri Lamb
Tucson, Arizona
November 1, 2013

Chapter 1

Care Coordination, Quality, and Nursing

Gerri Lamb, PhD, RN, FAAN

Care coordination is a key ingredient in our national agenda for improving the quality and affordability of health care in the United States. In their 2013 Progress Report to Congress on the National Strategy for Quality Improvement in Health Care, the U.S. Health and Human Services Department stated:

> *Conscious patient-centered coordination of care not only improves the patient experience, it also leads to better long-term health outcomes, as demonstrated by fewer unnecessary trips to the hospital, fewer repeated tests, fewer conflicting prescriptions, and clearer advice about the best course of treatment.* USDHHS, 2013.

Numerous local, state, and federal initiatives are underway to promote care coordination. Emerging healthcare delivery models, like patient-centered medical homes and accountable care organizations, are being designed to operationalize it. New technologies are being developed to support its key elements like care planning and communication across providers and settings. In this chapter, we explore the reasons for care coordination's explosive entry onto the national quality scene. We look at current definitions of care coordination and a little of its history to set the stage for the chapters to follow. As you will see, nurses have played a significant role in the history of care coordination and have many opportunities to shape its future in practice and policy.

EVOLUTION OF THE NATIONAL QUALITY STRATEGY

The most recent call for better care coordination emerged from our national focus on improving the quality of health care. The impetus for the current national quality agenda began over a decade ago with the Institute of Medicine (IOM) report, *To Err is Human* (IOM, 2000) which stunned professionals and consumers alike with its estimates of the magnitude of medical errors in the United States. Although the healthcare community was well aware of the gaps in U.S. performance on health indicators, such as life expectancy and access to care, the IOM report was seen as a resounding call to action. With this report and *Crossing the Quality Chasm* (2001) that closely followed, a national blueprint for action was established. A new system was envisioned, one that would achieve the six aims of safe, effective, patient-centered, timely, efficient, and equitable health care.

The IOM and their vision for our healthcare system were soon followed by numerous local and national initiatives. The practice community was joined by the academic and research community to find new ways to teach and improve quality and safety. In 2003, the IOM issued its companion report on *Health Professions Education* that was followed by a national nursing initiative to develop and implement educational competencies for safe, high-quality nursing practice (Cronenwett et al., 2007). The competencies that emerged from the Quality and Safety Education for Nurses (QSEN) program are now firmly embedded in accreditation standards for undergraduate and graduate nursing programs. QSEN also contributed to the development of an academic–practice learning community in which sharing of tools and resources became commonplace. Similar movements emerged in other professions, including medicine, pharmacy, and public health and have led to much improved codification of quality and safety competencies for practice.

While these changes were being made in health professions education, the practice community also moved quickly to identify quality problems and to implement systematic quality improvement strategies. Many of the quality improvement systems that are in place today were developed and refined in response to the need to address issues uncovered in the IOM reports. Subsequently, the quality and safety movement received a significant boost from federally funded demonstrations and policy that recognized the need for and created incentives for innovation and improvements. The Center for Medicare and Medicaid Innovation, for example, is an important clearinghouse for exciting new developments to improve quality and safety. Our current pay-for-performance and value-based purchasing programs that reward improved quality and impose penalties for avoidable adverse outcomes, like readmissions or falls, represent a dramatic change in the way that health care is thought about and financed in the U.S.

The common agenda in all of these changes, reaching back more than a decade now is to improve the health of the American public, their experience in the healthcare system, and to make care more affordable—what we now refer to as our National Quality Strategy for Quality Improvement in Health Care (USDHHS, 2013). The National Quality Strategy was formally established as part of the Patient Protection and Affordable Care Act signed into law in 2010.

THE ROLE OF CARE COORDINATION IN IMPROVING QUALITY AND SAFETY

Care coordination is front and center in the national quality agenda. It is identified as one of the six priorities of the National Quality Strategy, along with safer care, patient engagement, effective prevention and treatment, best practices in healthy living, and the development of new healthcare delivery models. While care coordination had been recognized as key to achieving the goals for the healthcare system in the earlier IOM reports, its inclusion in the National Quality Strategy has focused considerable attention on how it is defined and measured, as well as provided new impetus for the funding and design of innovative and cost-effective care coordination practices.

Care coordination has been defined in many ways. It often is referred to as the "glue" of our healthcare system, the process that transpires between patients, families, and members of the healthcare team to organize care and assure that everyone and every service is aligned and working toward the same goals. Two of the most commonly cited definitions come from the Agency for Healthcare Research and Quality (AHRQ) (McDonald et al., 2010) and the National Quality Forum (NQF) (2006):

> Care coordination is the deliberate organization of patient care activities between two or more participants (including the patient) involved in a patient's care to facilitate the appropriate delivery of health services. Organizing care includes marshaling of personnel and other resources needed to carry out all required patient care activities and is often managed by the exchange of information among participants responsible for different aspects of care. (McDonald et al., 2010, p. 4).

> Care coordination is a function that helps ensure that the patient's needs and preferences for health services and information sharing across people, functions, and sites are met over time. (NQF, 2006).

Both of these definitions emphasize that care coordination involves attending to the needs and preferences of patients and their families. The work of care coordination occurs at the intersection of patients, providers, and healthcare settings and relies on integrative activities including communication and mobilization of appropriate people and resources. It serves to connect the pieces and parts of health care to make it coherent and manageable for patients and providers alike. For many patients and their families, the experience of care coordination is equated with the effective relay of information between providers and across settings, less repetition of information and tests, and more timely and effective implementation of needed services (see the following box).

Think about the last time you, a family member, or a friend interacted with some part of the healthcare system. It might have been a visit with a primary care provider or a specialist or a trip to urgent care or the emergency room. It may have been a hospital admission, a stay in a nursing home, or a visit from home care or hospice in your home. You or your family member or friend may have been seen by a nurse, a physician, a therapist, a community worker, or another provider. Picture the encounter and what stands out for you as you recall this experience. How much of what you remember is related to effective care coordination as defined in the text?

These two definitions and most others speak to the common attributes of care coordination required by all individuals receiving health care. The expectation is that all patients, regardless of their diagnoses, the severity of their illnesses, or their social situation, need to have their care coordinated. All patients require that their providers address their needs and preferences, communicate pertinent information with other providers and across settings, and assure that needed treatments and services are implemented in a timely and effective way. Transitional care, the processes involved in linking care across settings, is an important component of care coordination for all patients. The definitions also allow room for the practice of more intense or extensive care coordination, frequently referred to as case management. Case management usually is reserved for individuals with a complex array of physical, emotional, and social health needs at risk of significant adverse outcomes and very expensive care. The relationship among care coordination, transitional care, and case management is shown in Figure 1.

Care coordination and its more intense version, case management, are not new to our healthcare system. Many different models have been developed and tested over a span of more than 50 years. Elements of today's care coordination programs can be found in federal demonstrations dating back to the 1970s and 1980s (Kemper, Applebaum, & Harrigan, 1987; Lamb, 2005). Care coordination and case management models emerged and often faded away according to national priorities and financing of the times. For instance, care coordination programs to assist frail elderly to remain in the community were initiated in the 1970s as federal demonstrations to reduce nursing home placements (Kemper, Applebaum, & Harrigan, 1986). In the late 1980s, 1990s, and later, numerous care coordination and case management programs were integrated into managed care plans and contracts to increase primary prevention and reduce expensive hospitalizations (Coleman et al., 2004; Naylor et al., 1999). The Community Nursing Organization (CNO) demonstration, one of the first tests of a nurse-led model of care coordination

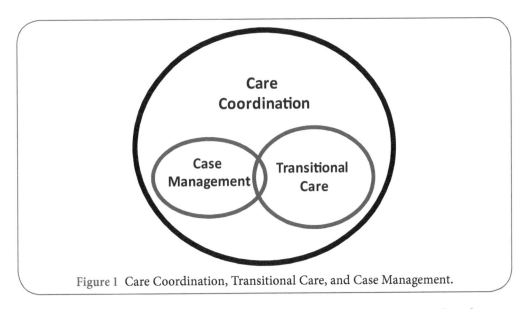

Figure 1 Care Coordination, Transitional Care, and Case Management.

and case management for Medicare beneficiaries, started in the early 1990s (Lamb, 1996; Schrader, Shelton, Britt, & Buttitta, 1996). One of the primary goals that the federal government had for initiating the CNOs was to reduce the overall utilization of emergency rooms and hospitals and escalating costs. The CNO model was consistent with the managed care framework which was gaining in popularity at the time.

Today's emphasis on care coordination and the emerging models, like these earlier ones, are a reflection of where we are in health care today and current priorities. The National Quality Strategy with its focus on improving quality and reducing costs incorporates many of the same themes that drove the development of previous care coordination models. Thus, we see a renewed emphasis, for instance, on reducing hospital readmissions and costs and population-based care for high-risk populations like people with heart failure or diabetes. Many of the core elements of care coordination practice that you will read about in the chapters to follow emerged during earlier cycles of care coordination and have been revised to meet the needs of the present practice and economic environment.

There are some important differences between today's care coordination models and those of the past. Certainly, the emergence of new technologies that support communication and standardized documentation has had a significant influence on care coordination practice. National policies that emphasize the importance of patient-centered care and the use of meaningful data in practice settings align closely with the needs and goals of effective care coordination. Today's emphasis on value and the demand to demonstrate systematic processes and their impact has led to numerous national initiatives to develop and implement clinical performance measures and public reporting relevant to care coordination. As a result, we now have a growing set of standardized measures for the processes and outcomes of care coordination (McDonald et al., 2010; NQF, 2010). New patient-centered measures of care coordination are also being developed.

Perhaps the greatest difference between today's care coordination and that of the past is the scope of interest in it and the extent of implementation. As noted earlier and emphasized throughout this book, care coordination has been identified as a major national strategy for achieving quality and cost outcomes. It is embedded in national policy related to the development of new practice arrangements and models, including accountable care organizations and patient-centered medical homes. It is recognized as a key intervention in value-based purchasing initiatives that incentivize healthcare systems for improved outcomes, such as reducing preventable hospitalizations or infections. Today's models of care coordination are intended for all people who use the healthcare system. Recognition of the need for care coordination for all individuals and a more intense level of care coordination, e.g., case management, for at-risk, vulnerable populations is not new. Almost all of the care coordination models that predate the ones we see today included a tiered approach to care coordination with different types and amount of interventions according to patient need and risk for adverse outcomes. What is different today is that these models are being implemented across all settings from primary care to hospital to long-term care and in the community. What those of us who were working in local or regional demonstrations and programs in the 1980s and 1990s envisioned for care coordination is now underway and supported by new practice models, technology, and methods and tools for evaluation.

CARE COORDINATION AND NURSES

Nurses have been central to the evolution of care coordination practice and to its many current iterations. The imprint and influence of nurses may be found on almost every care coordination model and intervention we see today. Nurses developed a number of the models you will read about in this book. They have crafted and refined many of the care coordination activities we see integrated into current programs to improve quality and safety. The close link between nursing and care coordination practice is reflected in *The Future of Nursing* "Coordinating care is one of the traditional strengths of the nursing profession, whether in the community or the acute care setting" (IOM, 2010, p. 65). The challenge for each of us today is to capitalize on the lessons of an extraordinary past and to use our considerable collective wisdom and knowledge about care coordination to make a difference in improving quality and reducing costs of health care. This work is happening right now at all levels of practice, education, research, and policy. It is more than likely going on at your university or practice institution (see "Where is care coordination happening around you" box).

The challenges facing those of us who want to improve care coordination and demonstrate its value to improving quality and reducing costs are well delineated in its extensive and still growing literature. Foundational issues, such as those concerned with clear operational definitions of interventions or sound measurement of care coordination, were identified early on and continue to be the focus of considerable work in nursing and our healthcare and policy communities. American Nurses Association's (ANA) current task force on care coordination, for example, is working on a framework that will guide future measure development and capture of data important to nursing's contributions to care

Where is care coordination happening around you?

Throughout this book, you will read over and over again that care coordination is pivotal to the national health and quality goals. What are the signs that this is happening? Where can you look around you to find care coordination in education, practice, or policy? Once you start asking questions, you are likely to find its footprints everywhere. You will find clues to answering these questions in the following chapters.

- What care coordination activities are going on in my practice setting?
- Are there people here who specialize in care coordination? What do they do?
- Am I doing care coordination?
- How is care coordination incorporated into nursing competencies and accreditation standards?
- Are the educational programs at my university or those in the local vicinity incorporating care coordination in the curriculum? Do we have any certificate or degree programs preparing nurses for care coordination, transitional care, or case management? Are new programs being planned?
- What are local researchers doing in the area of care coordination? What quality and cost outcomes are they looking at?
- What practices are being evaluated in academic programs or in healthcare settings that could be related to care coordination? How are people deciding whether their care coordination interventions are effective?
- Are there any new practice models starting up locally? Is care coordination included? Who's doing it? Who's paying for it?

coordination (ANA, 2012, 2013). Working at the policy level, the Nursing Alliance for Quality Care (NAQC) and the American Academy of Nursing (AAN) both have developed policy statements to guide research and funding priorities (NAQC, 2013; Cipriano, 2012). Many nurses are members and leaders of national workgroups and initiatives on care coordination practice, measurement, and policy. You will see the story and results of their efforts in the pages of this book.

As emphasized earlier in this chapter, the context for improving care coordination and demonstrating its impact is changing rapidly. We cannot and should not underestimate the power of technology and funding incentives to transform what is currently understood and valued about care coordination into something new and potentially unrecognizable. There are very real opportunities and threats when a highly valued, yet largely unrecognized practice, such as care coordination, reaches national attention. The experience may be very like that of an actor who has been toiling for years and finally has a break-through movie and finds him or herself in the national spotlight. There will be many who want to become part of the actor's—or, in this case, care coordination's—entourage because they believe in its value and impact and possibly many who see it as an opportunity for entrepreneurship and funding. All of this attention and movement are a natural part of growth and innovation.

The message of this book—and one that will be repeated sometimes implicitly, sometimes explicitly—is that nurses have the critical history, knowledge, and expertise needed to assure that care coordination achieves the goals set forth for it in the national quality agenda. We have a stake in making sure that the values, knowledge, and skills—all that define nursing competence in care coordination—come to the national practice, research, and policy tables to improve health care for our nation. This is not a story about ownership. Care coordination at its core is about effective communication, collaboration, and teamwork with patients, families, and all of the other members of the teams with whom we work. And as with all good teams, each and every member is responsible for contributing unique expertise that will make the whole better. For health care, it is critical that nurses understand – and use – and evaluate – and continue to innovate their care coordination expertise. All of this is essential as we work for the healthcare system that we want and need.

REFERENCES

American Nurses Association (ANA). (2012). Position statement: Care coordination and registered nurses' essential role. Retrieved from http://www.nursingworld.org/position/care-coordination.aspx

American Association (ANA). (2013). Care coordination quality measurement panel steering committee. Retrieved from http://www.nursingworld.org/MainMenuCategories/Policy-Advocacy/Professional-Issues-Panels/Care-Coordination-Quality-Measures-Panel

Cipriano, P. (2012). The imperative for patient, family, and population-centered interprofessional approaches to care coordination and transitional care: A policy brief by the American Academy of Nursing's Care Coordination Task Force. *Nursing Outlook, 60*(5), 330–333.

Coleman, E. A., Smith, J. D., Frank, J. C., Min, S., Parry, C., & Kramer, A. M. (2004). Preparing patients and caregivers to participate in care delivered across settings: The care transitions intervention. *Journal of the American Geriatrics Society, 52,* 1817–1825.

Cronenwett, L., Sherwood, G., Barnsteiner, J., Disch, J., Johnson., J., Mitchell, P., … Warren, J. (2007). Quality and safety education for nurses. *Nursing Outlook, 55*(3). 122–131.

Institute of Medicine (IOM). (2000). *To err is human: Building a safer health system.* Washington, DC: National Academies Press.

Institute of Medicine (IOM). (2001). *Crossing the quality chasm; A new health system for the 21st century.* Washington D.C.: National Academies Press.

Institute of Medicine (IOM). (2003). *Health professions education: A bridge to quality.* Washington, DC: National Academies Press.

Institute of Medicine (IOM). (2010). *The future of nursing: Leading change, advancing health.* Washington, D.C.: The National Academies Press.

Kemper, P., Applebaum, R., & Harrigan, M. (1987). Community demonstrations: What have we learned? *Health Care Financing Review, 8,* 87–100.

Lamb, G. (1995). Early lessons from a capitated community-based nursing model. *Nursing Administration Quarterly, 19*(3), 18–26.

Lamb, G. (1996). Case management. *Annual Review of Nursing Research, 13,* 117–136.

McDonald, K. M., Schultz, E., Albin, L., Pineda, N., Lonhard, J., Sundaram, C., … Malcolm, E. (2010). *Care coordination atlas version 3* (Prepared by Stanford University under subcontract to Battelle on Contract No. 290-04-0020). AHRQ Publication No: 11-0023-EF. Rockville, MD: Agency for Research and Quality.

National Quality Forum (NQF). (2006). *NQF-endorsed definition and framework for measuring and reporting care coordination.* Washington, D.C.: Author.

National Quality Forum (NQF). (2010). *Preferred practices and performance measures for measuring and reporting care coordination: A consensus report.* Washington, D.C.: Author.

Naylor, M. D., Brooten, D., Campbell, R., Jacobsen, B. S., Mezey, M. D., Pauly, M. V., & Schwartz, J. S. (1999). Comprehensive discharge planning and home follow-up of hospitalized elders: A randomized clinical trial. *Journal of the American Medical Association, 281,* 613–620.

Naylor, M. D. (2012). Advancing high value transitional care: The central role of nursing and its leadership. *Nursing Administration Quarterly April/June, 36*(2), 115–126.

Nursing Alliance for Quality Care (NAQC). The role of nurses in accountable care organizations: Information for policy-makers. Retrieved from http://www.naqc.org/Main/Resources/Publications/NursesRole-AccountableCareOrg.pdf

Samal L., Dykes P. C., Greenberg J., Hasan O., Venkatesh A. K., Volk. A., & Bates, D. W. (2012). *Environmental analysis of health information technology to support care coordination and care transitions.* Washington, DC: NQF.

Schraeder, C., & Shelton, P. (2011). *Comprehensive care coordination for chronically ill adults.* West Sussex, U.K.: John Wiley & Sons.

Schraeder, C., Shelton, P., Britt, T., & Buttitta, K. (1996). Case management in a capitated system: The community nursing organization. *Journal of Case Management,* 5(2), 58–64.

United States Department of Health and Human Services (USDHH). (2013). 2013 annual progress report to Congress: National strategy for quality improvement in health care. Retrieved from http://www.ahrq.gov/workingforquality/nqs/nqs2013annlrpt.htm

Section 1

Quality and Safety: The Foundation of Care Coordination Practice

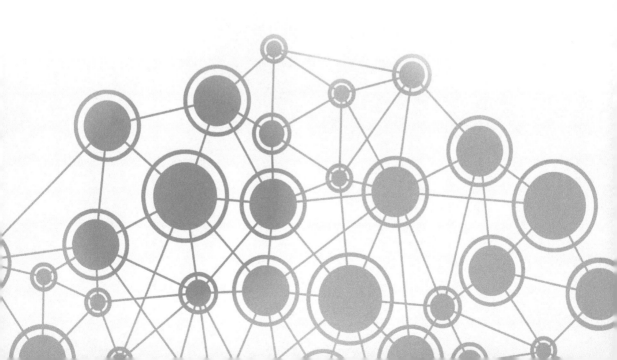

Chapter 2

Nursing and Quality: A Historical Perspective

Gail Armstrong, DNP, PhD(c), ACNS-BC, CNE

The National Strategy for Quality Improvement in Health Care (also known as the National Quality Strategy; http://www.ahrq.gov/workingforquality/) sets forth ambitious goals for improving the quality of health care in the United States. Established as part of the Patient Protection and Affordable Care Act of 2010, the National Quality Strategy builds on a long and rich tradition of quality improvement and innovation in nursing and health care. Nursing's many initiatives to educate nurses about quality improvement, implement evidence-based practice improvements, and measure nursing's contributions to quality and safety outcomes are closely woven together with key reports and events that anticipated and shaped today's quality agenda. This chapter describes several of the landmarks that paved the way to our National Quality Strategy and programs that have prepared nurses to play a central role in its implementation. Each of these landmarks and programs discussed in this chapter—and many others— have created the foundation for nurses to deliver on the promise of care coordination.

A QUALITY CHASM

Much of the precedent for today's National Quality Strategy was established with the Institute of Medicine's landmark report, *To Err is Human* (IOM, 2000). As noted in Chapter 1, this report quantified the magnitude of medical errors in the United States and precipitated intense scrutiny of current healthcare delivery and its outcomes. It set the stage for envisioning goals for a new healthcare system for the 21st century (IOM, 2001). While considerable attention was focused on the findings of *To Err is Human*, there were a number of studies that led up to this report. The Harvard Practice Study (Brennan, 1991; Leape, 1991) had a significant influence on the focus and goals of the

IOM report. Spurred by the upsurge of medical malpractice cases in the 1980s, the Harvard Practice Study was conducted by a group of researchers and clinicians who reviewed medical records of 30,000 patients in hospitals in New York. They found that 3.7% of these patients suffered an adverse event, defined as an injury caused by medical treatment, which either interrupted discharge or caused measurable harm. Of these events, 14% were fatal. Most strikingly, the authors estimated that approximately two-thirds of the adverse events were preventable (Brennan, 1991).

Following the Harvard Practice Study, Lucian Leape, published "Error in Medicine," an article that examined the pervasive nature of errors in health care. Leape (1994) described errors in health care as being equivalent to "system failures" and advocated for system-based improvements. These themes would figure prominently in each of the subsequent IOM Quality Chasm reports.

During the 1990s, more and more health organizations began to collect and analyze error rates. Concurrently in nursing, ANA started collecting nursing-specific data in 1998 to explore the relationship between nursing care and patient outcomes. Demonstration of nursing's contribution to important quality and patient outcomes—and value to health and healthcare delivery—became a central goal for the nursing community and a priority for nurse scientists and their interprofessional research teams. We will explore this later in the chapter when we look at initiatives designed to measure and report quality outcomes associated with quality nursing care.

IOM Reports on Quality and Safety

Between 2000 and 2006, the IOM published a series of 11 major reports focusing on documenting problems and recommending improvements to the U.S. healthcare system. The first report, *To Err Is Human*, shaped the goals and content of the subsequent reports by identifying glaring chasms in the U.S. healthcare system around safety, timeliness, efficiency, effectiveness, equity, patient-centeredness, and quality. Table 1 lists these 11 reports and their areas of emphasis. Their recommendations have had significant influence on trends in health systems research and quality improvement and are readily identifiable in a variety of emerging professional standards.

NURSING'S HISTORY OF HEALTHCARE QUALITY AND SAFETY

Nursing's concern about and attention to quality and safety long predate the surge of national interest initiated by the IOM reports. In the 19th century, Florence Nightingale emphasized the importance of keeping patients safe with her oft-quoted words: "It may seem a strange principle to enunciate as the very first requirement in a hospital that it

Table 1 Institute of Medicine's Quality Chasm Reports

IOM Report	Date Published	Focal Point
To Err Is Human	2000	There are 48,000 to 98,000 preventable deaths each year in U.S. hospitals due to medical errors and system failures.
Crossing the Quality Chasm	2001	The U.S. healthcare system needs to become increasingly safe, timely, efficient, equitable, effective, and patient-centered.
Leadership by Example: Coordinating Government Roles in Improving Health Care Quality	2002	The federal government can leverage its unique position as regulator, purchaser, provider, and research sponsor to improve care—not only in the six major healthcare programs in the report that serve almost 100 million people, but also throughout the nation's healthcare system.
Fostering Rapid Advances in Health Care: Learning from Systems Demonstrations	2002	Lessons for improving quality and safety should be gleaned from current practice innovations. New demonstrations are needed to provide models for health system reform.
Priority Areas for National Action: Transforming Health Care Quality	2003	The U.S. Department of Health and Human Services (DHHS) and other groups in the public and private sectors should focus on an identified set of 20 priority areas to improve the quality of health care delivered to all Americans. These priority areas represent the spectrum of health care from preventive care to end-of-life care. They also touch on all age groups, healthcare settings, and healthcare providers.
Health Professions Education: A Bridge to Quality	2003	Students of all health professions need to be educated in providing care that employs patient-centeredness, quality improvement, evidence-based practice, teamwork and collaboration, and informatics.
Patient Safety: Achieving a New Standard for Care	2003	The United States requires a detailed plan to facilitate the development of data standards applicable to the collection, coding, and classification of patient safety information. Key areas related to the establishment of a national health information infrastructure are identified.
Keeping Patients Safe: Transforming the Work Environment of Nurses	2004	The characteristics of the work environment in which patient care is provided may have significant impact on quality and safety. As the largest component of the healthcare workforce, nurses require work environments that promote safe practices and effective outcomes.
Quality Through Collaboration: The Future of Rural Health Care	2004	There is a dearth of research on the quality of rural health care. The recommendations from previous IOM reports need to be tailored for the rural healthcare setting.
Preventing Medication Errors	2006	Medication errors are common and costly. This report outlines a comprehensive approach to decreasing the prevalence of these errors by engaging patients, families, healthcare providers and organizations, and government agencies.
Improving the Quality of Health Care for Mental and Substance-Use Conditions	2006	This report examines the extent to which approaches and solutions proposed in the Quality Chasm series are applicable to mental health and substance-use services. A comprehensive strategy for integration of mental health, substance use, and other healthcare services is proposed.

should do the sick no harm" (Nightingale, 1992). Nightingale also endorsed standard procedures and reliable processes as vital to improving patient outcomes. She anticipated the core principles of today's quality improvement processes as well as a dramatic shift to system accountability for quality.

> Let whoever is in charge, keep this simple question in her head (not, how can I always do the right thing myself), but how can I provide for this right thing to be always done? ....the pride is rather in carrying on a system....
>
> Nightingale, 1992, 6.

Nursing's commitment to quality and safety were recognized and advanced in a number of the IOM reports, especially *Keeping Patients Safe* (2004), which focused on the pivotal role of the nursing workforce in safeguarding quality. Several of the IOM reports provided the impetus to explore nursing education and competencies for quality practice and provided the framework for engaging nurses in quality improvement. Two initiatives, Quality and Safety Education for Nurses and Transforming Care at the Bedside, both funded by The Robert Wood Johnson Foundation (RWJF), accelerated nursing preparation and participation in quality improvement.

Quality and Safety Education for Nurses (QSEN)

The Quality and Safety Education for Nurses (QSEN) initiative has educated thousands of nursing faculty about quality and safety competencies and innovative ways to prepare students to achieve them. QSEN was developed in response to IOM's 2003 *Health Professions Education* report that recommended that all health professions students be educated in patient-centered care, evidence-based practice, quality improvement, teamwork and collaboration, and informatics. The steering committee that worked on the QSEN competencies added safety as a sixth essential competency for nursing students noting that nurses are uniquely positioned to protect patient safety (Cronenwett et al., 2007).

QSEN's thought leaders developed definitions for the six competencies; these definitions are outlined in Table 2. Additionally, the faculty of QSEN explicated the necessary knowledge, skills, and attitudes (KSAs) to operationalize each of the six competencies. These are available at QSEN's website: www.qsen.org. Also available on QSEN's website are peer-reviewed teaching strategies for those who teach health professions students, as well as various types of resources useful for nurses in all clinical settings.

Table 2 Quality and Safety Education for Nurses (QSEN) Competencies with Definitions

Competency	QSEN Definition
Patient-centered care	Recognize the patient as a full partner and the source of control in providing compassionate, coordinated care based on the patient's preferences, values, and needs.
Teamwork and collaboration	Function within nursing and interprofessional teams, fostering open communication, mutual respect, shared decision-making for quality patient care.
Evidence-based practice	Integrate best current evidence with clinical expertise, patient/family preferences and values for delivery of optimal health care.
Quality improvement	Use data to monitor care processes outcomes and employ improvement methods to design and test changes to continuously improve the quality and safety of healthcare systems.
Safety	Minimizes risk of harm to patients and providers through system effectiveness, individual performance.
Informatics	Use information and technology for communication, knowledge management, error mitigation, and decision-making support.

Source: Adapted from Cronenwett et al., 2007

Transforming Care at the Bedside (TCAB)

Transforming Care at the Bedside (TCAB) was a national strategic program also funded by the RWJF to invite bedside nurses' participation to make inpatient care safer, more reliable, more patient-centered, and to increase the vitality of the work environment (Buerhaus, 2011). Initiated in 2003, another important goal of TCAB was to increase satisfaction of the nurses providing care at the bedside on medical–surgical units. Early in its work, TCAB was a cooperative initiative between the Institute for Healthcare Improvement (IHI) and RWJF. IHI provided early leadership for TCAB bringing three hospitals into a pilot program that later expanded to 13 hospitals. The American Organization of Nurse Executives (AONE) became a third partner and has continued the work of TCAB through a learning cooperative with hospitals around the country.

The standardized framework for TCAB units was to develop an improvement project in one of four categories: 1) safe and reliable care, 2) vitality and teamwork, 3) patient-centered care, and 4) value-added processes. During the TCAB initiative, hospitals tested, refined, and implemented improvement concepts. Exemplar projects included: use of rapid response teams to "rescue" patients before a crisis occurs; models that support consistent and clear communication among caregivers; professional support programs such as preceptorships and educational opportunities; innovative diet plans and meal schedules for patients; and redesigned workspaces that enhance efficiency and limit waste (IHI, n.d).

TCAB piloted numerous tools and strategies to encourage active engagement of bedside nurses in quality improvement. The nurses were provided with a set of five core questions (Table 3) to ask their managers about participation in quality initiatives. The questions addressed several of the common concerns about generating and executing quality improvement work on nursing units, such as the availability of training and resources as well as the opportunity to have an active voice in the projects. The dialogue between bedside nurses and managers helped to anticipate key obstacles and to build sustainability of the quality improvement programs.

The essence of TCAB was to create opportunities to fast track nursing's contributions to quality and safety innovations through nurse-led testing, assessing, and implementing of care improvement strategies. The 10 hospitals that continued through IHI's four-year initiative tested 426 different rapid cycle change projects in the first two years, and implemented and sustained approximately 284 care improvements (Buerhaus, 2011). Additionally, analysis indicated that on average, TCAB units had fewer patient falls with harm and less RN turnover and overtime compared with other hospitals in the U.S. (Unruh, Agrawal, & Hassmiller, 2011). Cost/benefit analysis calculated from these 10 units between 2004 and 2007 was a benefit of more than $625,000/unit (Unruh et al., 2011). TCAB not only demonstrated the insight that bedside clinicians possess in terms of identifying and implementing effective unit-based quality improvement initiatives, but it also quantified the cost effectiveness of these initiatives.

Table 3 Core Questions of the Transforming Care at the Bedside (TCAB) Initiative

Core Questions of the Transforming Care at the Bedside (TCAB) Initiative	
1	"What are you asking me to do?"
2	"What is in it for me?" "What is in it for my patient?"
3	"You are telling us we are going to have a voice in control: can we trust you?"
4	"I don't have time to do my work now; where am I going to find time to do this?"
5	"I haven't been trained to do this, what help are you going to give me?"

Source: Buerhaus, 2011

Practice Standards and Models of Excellence

Quality and safety standards are codified for all nurses. The American Nurses Association (2010) specifies and provides exemplars for quality practice (Table 4). Nurses are expected to have the requisite knowledge, skills, and attitudes to carry out each of these functions related to quality improvement. Notice that the exemplars of competent practice are relevant across practice settings and incorporate key quality and safety outcomes.

Table 4 ANA Competencies Associated wth Quality of Practice with Clinical Exemplars

ANA Competency	Clinical Exemplar
Identifying aspects of practice important for quality monitoring	Tracking length of stay, discharge, teaching needs, or fall rate over time
Using indicators to monitor quality, safety, and effectiveness of nursing practice	Tracking primary care office's readmissions to the hospital over a six month period
Collecting data to monitor quality and effectiveness of nursing practice	Tracking utilization of a checklist by healthcare teams to address all facets of a care bundle
Analyzing quality data to identify opportunities for improving nursing practice	Tracking post-discharge patient satisfaction data collected to identify areas for improvement
Formulating recommendations to improve nursing practice or outcomes	Updating clinical policies based on emerging evidence-based standards
Implementing activities to enhance the quality of nursing practice	Engaging in ongoing quality improvement work to improve patient and nurse satisfaction
Developing, implementing, and/or evaluating policies, procedures, and guidelines to improve the quality of practice.	Staying current with evidence-based best practices to update nursing unit standards
Participating on and/or leading efforts to minimize costs and unnecessary duplication	Working with process improvement experts to identify process waste in daily operations
Identifying problems that occur in day-to-day work routines in order to correct process inefficiencies	Organizing a task force to decrease waiting time between writing of discharge orders and patient's ability to leave hospital
Analyzing factors related to quality, safety and effectiveness	Identifying the between-appointment education needs of patients in a specialty clinic
Analyzing organizational systems for barriers to quality healthcare consumer outcomes	Organizing a task force to look at outdated policies that contribute to patient/family dissatisfaction (e.g., family visiting hours)
Implementing processes to remove or weaken barriers within organizational systems	Examining the research evidence and outcomes on allowing families or support people to stay at a patient's bedside, thereby eliminating visiting hours
Providing leadership in the design and implementation of quality improvements	Providing a cost comparison study on bundling supplies for common care interventions (e.g., insertion of a peripheral intravenous line)
Designing innovations to effect change in practice and improve health outcomes	Developing the use of home-based technologies to enhance home care nurses' abilities to support patients and monitor/trend data related to chronic conditions (e.g., BP, blood sugars, weight)
Evaluating the practice environment and quality of nursing care rendered in relation to existing evidence	Reorganizing the physical environment of an inpatient nursing unit to decrease interruptions to nurses as they administer medications
Identifying opportunities for the generation and use of research and evidence	Evaluating home care policies based on latest relevant evidence
Obtaining and maintaining professional certification if it is available in the area of expertise	Nurses can be certified in practice areas (e.g., medical/surgical nursing, palliative care, critical care nursing) or as advanced practice clinicians (e.g., nurse practitioners, clinical nurse specialists, nurse midwives)
Using the results of quality improvement to initiative changes in nursing practice and the healthcare delivery system	Conducting rapid cycle PDSA (plan, do, study, act) to evaluate patient fall outcomes in response to early identification of patients at risk for falls

Source: ANA, 2010

Emerging models of excellence supported by professional nursing organizations also have an explicit emphasis on quality and patient safety. The American Nurses Credentialing Center (ANCC), for example, was the driving force in developing the Magnet Recognition Program®, whose original work was to identify the operational elements of an acute care setting that effectively link nursing care, patient safety, and quality of care (Lundmark, 2008). Of the 27 goals recommended by the Institute of Medicine (IOM) in *Keeping Patients Safe: Transforming the Work Environment of the Nurse* (2004), 20 goals are addressed by required elements in the Magnet Recognition application and accreditation processes (Lundmark, 2008). Similarly, the American Academy of Nursing recognizes innovators in the development of effective delivery models in their Raise the Voice Edge Runners program (http://www.aannet.org/rtv_edgerunners). Many of the recipients of Edge Runner recognition developed care models and interventions that demonstrate the sustained clinical and financial impact of care coordination.

MOVING QUALITY FORWARD

Driven by the impetus created by the IOM reports and the national attention focused on improving quality, a groundswell of activities were initiated to embed standards and incentives for quality in regulatory guidelines, accreditation, and payment reform. Much of this has played out over the past decade and has been accelerated by the Patient Protection and Affordable Care Act. The array of activities undertaken to standardize and incentivize quality are extensive; a few examples are provided to illustrate the kinds of programs underway.

National Patient Safety Goals

Inclusion of patient safety practices in accreditation standards for healthcare organizations quickly advanced patient safety standards. In 2002, The Joint Commission initiated a program to establish National Patient Safety Goals (NPSGs) and introduced them into accreditation standards the following year. NPSGs are a series of specific actions that accredited organizations are required to include in their care to prevent common medical errors, such as miscommunication among caregivers, unsafe use of infusion pumps, and medication mix-ups.

Each of the patient safety goals is based on analysis of trends in national sentinel event data and recommendations of The Joint Commission's Patient Safety Advisory Group. The Advisory Group is composed of nurses, physicians, pharmacists, risk managers, clinical engineers, and other professionals who have hands-on experience in addressing patient safety issues in diverse healthcare settings. The goal for implementation of

NPSGs in accreditation standards is to promote systematic implementation of quality improvement programs in health facilities and to prevent and reduce serious medical errors and sentinel events. Recent studies of sentinel events show a rise in the number of reported events since 2004 (Health Reference Center Academic, 2012). Today, the majority of sentinel events are self-reported by facilities, which may be interpreted as a signal of widespread uptake of quality improvement initiatives and the recognition that sentinel events and errors require close monitoring and system solutions.

Translating Evidence into Practice

While there has been a long-standing emphasis on translating research findings for practice, the quality agenda provided a significant boost. Numerous public and private organizations have encouraged and funded initiatives to accelerate application of evidence into daily practice. One promising effort groups evidence-based strategies in intervention "bundles." Bundles are defined as "a small set of evidence-based interventions for a defined patient segment/population and care setting that when implemented together will result in significantly better outcomes than when implemented individually" (Resar, Griffin, Haraden, & Nolan, 2012, p. 2). The first initiative to create and test care bundles was in critical care; projects soon expanded to other hospital units and settings. Researchers found that by consistently using a small set of evidence-based interventions for defined patient populations' improvements in patient outcomes exceeded expectations.

Nurses are central to the development, use, and evaluation of care bundles. In his article on care bundles and the early pioneering work of Peter Pronovost, the recipient of an McArthur Genius Award, Atul Gawande shared the following story of Pronovost's first attempt to implement a standardized checklist for central line insertions:

> The next month, he and his team persuaded the hospital administration to authorize nurses to stop doctors if they saw them skipping a step on the checklist; nurses were also to ask them each day whether any lines ought to be removed, so as not to leave them in longer than necessary. This was revolutionary. Nurses have always had their ways of nudging a doctor into doing the right thing, ranging from the gentle reminder ("Um, did you forget to put on your mask, doctor?") to more forceful methods. (I've had a nurse body check me when she thought I hadn't put enough drapes on a patient.) But many nurses aren't sure whether this is their place, or whether a given step is worth a confrontation. (Does it really matter whether a patient's legs are draped for a line going into the chest?) The new rule made it clear: if doctors didn't follow every step on the checklist, the nurses would have backup from the administration to intervene. (Gawande, 2007).

The first care bundles were developed to reduce ventilator associated complications and central venous line infections. Most of the steps in the ventilator bundle—elevation of the head of the bed, assessment of readiness to extubate, prophylactic treatment of peptic ulcer disease and deep vein thrombosis and daily oral care with chlorhexadine—are carried out or overseen by nurses in collaboration with physicians and members of the care team. This also is the case for steps in the central line bundle (Resar et al, 2012). Introduction of care bundles is a successful example of the efficient use of evidence-based practices to improve quality. Teamwork is critical in the implementation of bundles, and nurses are at the center of this coordination.

Never Events and Payment Incentives

Recent changes in reimbursement strategies by the Centers for Medicare and Medicaid Services (CMS) have played an important role in advancing quality initiatives and patient safety standards. Beginning in October 2008, CMS announced that it would no longer reimburse for care associated with eight hospital-acquired conditions (HAC). The 2008 policy requires that hospitals report on the presence of these eight conditions at admission to clearly identify whether the condition developed during a hospitalization. Beginning in 2008, Medicare denied payment for hospital costs of treating the following conditions that may occur while a patient is in the hospital: Stage III or IV pressure ulcer; falls and trauma; surgical site infection after bariatric surgery, certain orthopedic procedures, and bypass surgery; central line-associated bloodstream infections; catheter-associated urinary tract infections; administration of incompatible blood; an air embolism; and a foreign object unintentionally retained after surgery (Straube, 2009). We can anticipate further alignment of payment strategies and safety and quality performance as we move forward in establishing a patient-centered and value-based healthcare system.

THE IMPORTANCE OF QUALITY MEASUREMENT

Quality improvement efforts rely on being able to measure and document changes over time. Each of the major frameworks and approaches to quality improvement, such as Six Sigma or Lean, require initial measurement of outcomes followed by measurement of evidence-based interventions and post-intervention outcomes. Recognizing that improvement efforts were impeded by lack of standardization of quality measures, many organizations, including The Joint Commission and the Centers for Medicare and Medicaid Services embarked on long-term programs to establish standardized measure sets for performance improvement and public reporting. Today, standardized measures and measurement sets are used as part of accreditation processes for healthcare organizations and for pay-for-performance and value-based purchasing programs.

While there are still considerable gaps in quality measurement sets, including those for care coordination, there has been extraordinary progress in recent years. An extensive infrastructure now exists for soliciting measures from researchers and clinicians, for conducting systematic reviews of their performance, and for moving important and scientifically sound measures into practice. Many nurses lead and/or participate in national measurement standard workgroups and review panels.

Capturing Nursing Contributions to Quality Outcomes

Nursing has an important stake in assuring that measures used in performance evaluation and public reporting capture their contributions to patient outcomes. Numerous initiatives have contributed to a better understanding of the relationship between nursing interventions and quality outcomes, including patient falls, infection rates, and hospital readmission.

Early projects like the Patient Safety and Quality Initiative funded by the American Nurses Association established the foundation for the development of quality measures sensitive to the work of nurses and nursing interventions (Gallagher, 2003; Montalvo, 2007). These measures, called nurse-sensitive indicators, drew attention to nurses' contributions to highly visible quality outcomes, like falls or infections, and the structural and process variables that influence them. Examples from this early set of nurse-sensitive indicators that were incorporated into the National Database of Nursing Quality Indicators (NDNQI) are shown in Table 5.

Many of these indicators were evaluated and endorsed by the National Quality Forum, a nonprofit, public-service organization that reviews and endorses standardized healthcare measures (NQF, 2004, 2007). The initial set of nurse-sensitive measures endorsed by NQF is shown in Table 6. The measures for smoking cessation and nurse turnover were dropped from this endorsed list during subsequent review in NQF's regular review cycle.

These initial efforts at establishing standardized indicators for nursing practices and outcomes have expanded through their implementation in the American Nurses' Association's NDNQI and collaborative registry programs like the Collaborative Alliance for Nursing Outcomes (CALNOC, 2012). Hundreds of hospitals participate in the CALNOC database that provides facility-specific and group benchmarking data on nursing practice and outcomes. Initiatives to develop, test and gain endorsement of nurse-sensitive measures were critical to heightening awareness of nursing's contributions

Table 5 American Nurses' Association Nurse-Sensitive
Indicators and Measures in the NDNQI® Database

Indicator	Sub-Indicator	Measure(s)
1. Nursing hours per patient day	a. Registered nurses (RNs)	Structure
	b. Licensed practical nurses (LPNs)/ Licensed vocational nurses (LVNs)	
	c. Unlicensed assistive personnel (UAP)	
2. Patient falls		Process and outcome
3. Patient falls with injury	a. Injury Level	Process and outcome
4. Pediatric pain assessment, intervention, reassessment (AIR) cycle		Process
5. Pediatric peripheral intravenous infiltration rate		Outcome
6. Pressure ulcer prevalence	a. Community acquired	Process and outcome
	b. Hospital acquired	
	c. Unit acquired	
7. Psychiatric physical/sexual assault rate		Outcome
8. Restraint prevalence		Outcome
9. RN education/certification		Structure
10. RN satisfaction survey option	a. Job satisfaction scales	Process and outcome
	b. Job satisfaction scales— Short form	
11. Skill mix: percent of total nursing hours supplied by:	a. RNs	Structure
	b. LPNs/LVNs	
	c. UAP	
	d. % of total nursing hours supplied by agency staff	
12. Voluntary nurse turnover		Structure
13. Nurse vacancy rate		Structure
14. Nosocomial infections	a. Urinary catheter-associated urinary tract infection	Outcome
	b. Central line catheter-associated blood stream infection (CLABSI)	
	c. Ventilator-associated pneumonia	

Table 6 National Quality Forum's 15 Nurse-Sensitive Measures

NQF Indicator	Definition
Death among surgical inpatients with treatable serious complications (failure to rescue):	The percentage of major surgical inpatients who experience a hospital-acquired complication and die.
Pressure ulcer prevalence:	Percentage of inpatients who have a hospital acquired pressure ulcer.
Falls prevalence	Number of inpatient falls per inpatient days.
Falls with injury	Number of inpatient falls with injuries per inpatient days.
Restraint prevalence	Percentage of inpatients who have a vest or limb restraint.
Catheter-associated UTI	Rate of urinary tract infections associated with use of urinary catheters for ICU patients.
Central line catheter-associated blood stream infection rate for ICU and high-risk nursery patients	Rate of blood stream infections associated with use of central line catheters for ICU and high-risk nursery patients.
Ventilator-associated pneumonia for ICU and high-risk nursery patients	Rate of pneumonia associated with use of ventilators for ICU and high-risk nursery patients.
Smoking cessation counseling for acute myocardial infarction.	
Smoking cessation counseling for heart failure.	
Smoking cessation counseling for pneumonia.	
Skill mix	Percentage of registered nurse, licensed vocational/practical nurse, unlicensed assistive personnel, and contracted nurse care hours to total nursing care hours.
Nursing care hours per patient day	Number of registered nurses per patient day and number of nursing staff hours (registered nurse, licensed vocational/practical nurse, and unlicensed assistive personnel) per patient day
Practice Environment Scale—Nursing Work Index	Composite score and scores for five subscales: 1. Nurse participation in hospital affairs 2. Nursing foundations for quality of care 3. Nurse manager ability, leadership, and support of nurses 4. Staffing and resource adequacy 5. Collegiality of nurse–physician relations.
Voluntary turnover	Number of voluntary uncontrolled separations during the month by category (RNs, APNs, LVN/LPNs, NAs).

Source: NQF, 2004

to quality and safety. Today, there is less emphasis on nurse-specific or profession-specific measures as we move to patient-centered, team-based measures. Much of the earlier work prepared nurses and the nursing community to be active participants in numerous current initiatives to align existing and new measures with the National Quality Strategy.

THE FUTURE OF QUALITY AND SAFETY THROUGH CARE COORDINATION

As is evident in this chapter's brief review of important developments in quality improvement in health care, there have been impressive gains over the past decade. Nursing has made major contributions to this progress. The authors of *The Future of Nursing* (IOM, 2010) explain below why nurses will play a significant role in the changes ahead:

> Nursing practice covers a broad continuum from health promotion, to disease prevention, to coordination of care, to cure—when possible—and to palliative care when cure is not possible. This continuum of practice is well matched to the current and future needs of the American people. Nurses have a direct effect on patient care. They provide the majority of patient assessments, evaluations, and care in hospitals, nursing homes, clinics, schools, workplaces, and ambulatory settings. They are at the front lines in ensuring that care is delivered safely, effectively, and compassionately. Additionally, nurses attend to parents and families in a holistic way that often goes beyond physical health needs to recognize and respond to social, mental, and spiritual needs. Given their education, experience, and unique perspectives and the centrality of their role providing care, nurses will play a significant role in the transformation of the healthcare system. (IOM, 2010, p. 23–24).

Each of the people and events described in this chapter—Florence Nightingale, the influential IOM reports, the initiatives to measure and reward quality care and outcomes— all have been important in setting the stage for our current National Quality Strategy and its far-reaching agenda to transform our healthcare system. The practice and study of care coordination is embedded in many of these reports and initiatives. Today's National Quality Strategy encompasses what we have learned about quality and how to integrate it in education and practice and to use it as a guide for setting national priorities for research and innovation. Importantly, the National Quality Strategy recognizes the work of care coordination as pivotal to achieving national quality goals. As you will read in the chapters that follow, care coordination is deeply embedded in nursing's history and practice and one of its major contributions to revolutionizing quality care.

REFERENCES

American Nurses Association (ANA). (2010). *Nursing: Scope and standards of practice* (2nd ed.). Silver Spring, MD: Nursebooks.org.

American Nurses Association (ANA). (n.d.) About NDNQI. Retrieved from http://www.nursingquality.org/

Beck, S. L., Weiss, M. E., Ryan-Wenger, N., Donaldson, N. E., Aydin, C., Towsley, G. L., et al. (2013). Measuring nurses' impact on health care quality: Progress, challenges, and future directions. *Medical Care,51*, S15–S22.

Brennan, T. A. (2004). Incidence of adverse events and negligence in hospitalized patients: Results of the Harvard Medical Practice Study I. 1991. *Quality & Safety in Health Care, 13*(2), 145–51; discussion 151.

Buerhaus, P. J. (2011). Lessons from TCAB, and more: An interview with health economist and quality researcher Jack Needleman. *Nursing Economics, 28*(4), 276–286.

Collaborative Alliance for Nursing Outcomes (CALNOC). (2012). Medication administration standards 2012: Measure definitions and coding instructions. Retrieved from www.calnoc.org

Cronenwett, L., Sherwood, G., Barnsteiner, J., Disch, J., Johnson, J., Mitchell, P., et al. (2007). Quality and safety education for nurses. *Nursing Outlook, 55*(3), 122–131.

Dossey, B. M. (2010). Florence Nightingale's vision for health and healing. *Journal of Holistic Nursing, 28*(4), 221–224.

Gallagher, R. M. (2003). Claiming the future of nursing through nursing-sensitive quality indicators. *Nursing Administration Quarterly, 27*(4), 273–284.

Gawande, A. (2007). The checklist. *The New Yorker*. Retrieved from http://www.newyorker.com/reporting/2007/12/10/071210fa_fact_gawande

Health Reference Center Academic. TJC releases sentinel events report. *Hospital Peer Review 37*(9), 97–108. Retrieved from http://www.ahcmedia.com/public/samples/hpr.pdf

Institute for Healthcare Improvement (n.d.). Transforming care at the bedside: Overview. Retrieved from http://www.ihi.org/offerings/initiatives/paststrategicinitiatives/tcab/Pages/default.aspx

Institute of Medicine (IOM). (2000). *To err is human: Building a safer health system* (1st ed.). J. M. Corrigan & M. S. Donaldson (Eds.). Washington, DC: National Academies Press.

Institute of Medicine (IOM). (2001). *Crossing the quality chasm: A new health system for the 21st century* (1st ed.). Washington, DC: National Academies Press.

Institute of Medicine (IOM). (2004). *Keeping patients safe: Transforming the work environment of nurses* (1st ed.). A. Page (Ed.). Washington, DC: National Academies Press.

Institute of Medicine (IOM). (2006). *Preventing medication errors: Quality chasm series* (1st ed.). P. Aspden, J. Wolcott, J. L. Bootman, & L. R. Cronenwett (Eds.). Washington, DC: National Academies Press.

The Joint Commission (TJC). (n.d.-a). Sentinel events. Retrieved from http://www.jointcommission.org/sentinel_event.aspx

The Joint Commission (TJC). (n.d.-b). Core measure sets. Retrieved from http://www.jointcommission.org/core_measure_sets.aspx

Leape, L. L. (1991). The nature of adverse events in hospitalized patients. Results of the Harvard Medical Practice Study II. *The New England Journal of Medicine, 324*(6), 377–384.

Leape, L. L. (1994). Error in medicine. *The Journal of the American Medical Association, 272*(23), 1851–1857.

Lundmark, V. (2008). Magnet environments for professional nursing practice – Patient safety and quality – NCBI Bookshelf. Retrieved from http://www.ncbi.nlm.nih.gov/books/NBK2667/

Montalvo, I. (2007). The national database of nursing quality indicators (NDNQI). *The Online Journal of Issues in Nursing, 12*. Retrieved from http://nursingworld.org/MainMenuCategories/ANAMarketplace/ANAPeriodicals/OJIN/TableofContents/Volume122007/No3Sept07/NursingQualityIndicators.html

National Quality Forum (NQF). (2004). *National voluntary consensus standards for nursing-sensitive care: An initial performance measure set*. Washington, DC: National Quality Forum. Retrieved from http://www.qualityforum.org/Publications/2004/10/National_Voluntary_Consensus_Standards_for_Nursing-Sensitive_Care__An_Initial_Performance_Measure_Set.aspx

National Quality Forum. (2007*). Tracking NQF-endorsed consensus standards for nursing-sensitive care: A 15-month study*. Washington, DC: National Quality Forum.

Nightingale, F. (1992). *Notes on Nursing* (1st ed.). Philadelphia, PA: Lippincott Williams & Wilkins.

Reason, J. (2000). Human error: models and management. *Western Journal of Medicine, 172*(6), 393–396.

Resar, R., Griffin, F.A., Haraden, C., & Nolan, T.W. (2012). Using care bundles to improve health care quality. IHI Innovation Series white paper. Cambridge, MA: Institute for Healthcare Improvement.

Straube, B. (2009). The policy on paying for treating hospital-acquired conditions: CMS officials respond. *Health Affairs, 28*(5), 1494–1497.

Unruh, L., Agrawal, M., & Hassmiller, S. (2011). The business case for Transforming Care at the Bedside among the TCAB 10 and lessons learned. *Nursing Administration Quarterly, 32*(2), 97–109.

Models and Tools for Improving Quality and Safety

Corrine Abraham, DNP, RN

T he national priorities for improving healthcare quality have provided an imperative to healthcare providers and a tremendous opportunity for the nursing profession to lead reform efforts as integral members of the healthcare team (AHRQ, n.d.). Nurses' commitment to patient- and family-centered care, paired with essential knowledge and skills in quality improvement (QI) methods lays the foundation for fully engaging in the national quality agenda. A plethora of practice guidelines and QI methods have been published and integrated into healthcare organizations to guide improvement efforts. Chapter 3 presents an overview of QI methods integrating illustrative examples of frameworks, tools, and resources for addressing challenges to improving quality. The Three Pillars of Quality Improvement model by Batalden and Davidoff (2007)—better system performance, better professional development, better patient and system outcomes—provides the overarching framework for the discussion. A number of sidebars provide short case examples, guided inquiry exercises, and exemplars to deepen understanding of QI.

OVERVIEW OF NURSE ROLE IN CONTINUOUS QUALITY IMPROVEMENT

Nurses are challenged to meet growing demands as they strive to coordinate care for clients with increasingly complex health needs while practicing at the fullest extent of their licenses. To promote quality care, the nurse must find a balance between endeavors that enhance health outcomes, professional development, and system performance. The Three Pillars of Quality Improvement model (Figure 1) (Batalden & Davidoff, 2007) illustrates that everyone has a responsibility for transforming healthcare. The model emphasizes that efforts to improve patient outcomes must be complemented by efforts to promote performance of the system, as well as development of the professional. Daily practice must incorporate implementation and evaluation of strategies focused on each of the pillars so that examination of professional and system performance, along with patient outcomes, becomes an integral part of the work of nurses, and not simply an add-on. Continuous quality improvement (CQI) requires developing and sustaining a habit of reflective practice—the cornerstone for continuous learning and adapting. Practice-based learning necessitates that nurses "connect their scientific knowledge to daily work patterns and embrace opportunities ... as they continually arise" (TJC, 2007, p. 1). Nurses have a tremendous opportunity to make significant contributions to promote CQI as a patient advocate, pivotal member of the healthcare team, care coordinator, leader in the clinical setting, and mentor for young professionals.

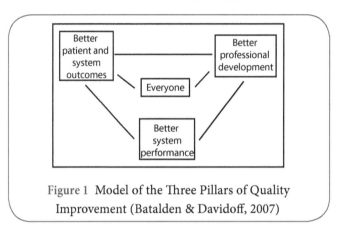

Figure 1 Model of the Three Pillars of Quality Improvement (Batalden & Davidoff, 2007)

BETTER SYSTEM PERFORMANCE

To understand system performance as one of the pillars for improvement, the nurse must understand the complexity of the health system, as well as the complexity of the problems encountered. Systems' thinking enables the nurse to coordinate care across different units and settings, adapting QI methods appropriately to meet the unique needs of each context. Thoughtful assessment of client characteristics, the practice setting, and interrelation with other collaborating or overarching systems creates the backbone for initiating and sustaining QI efforts.

The nurse must fully understand the surrounding political, economic, and social climate; the capabilities of the local health system; and the attributes, goals, and needs of the client to effectively advocate for clients in improving care. In the context of healthcare reform and national priorities, the National Quality Strategy has outlined three

> ### Case In Point
> As a clinical nurse leader in a large integrated health system, you have been asked to lead a new interprofessional committee on preventing falls and fall-related injury. As a relative newcomer, what do you need to understand about the context or system? What are possible drivers for the appointment of this committee? (Suggested answers at end of chapter)

aims—better care, healthy people and communities, and care that is affordable (USDHHS DHHS, 2011). In the acute care setting, the Transforming Care at the Bedside (TCAB) initiative discussed in Chapter 2 provides the context for engaging front-line staff and nurse managers in quality improvement, focusing on "safe and reliable care, vitality and teamwork, patient-centered care, value-added care processes" (AHRQ, 2011). A multitude of resources are available to guide improvements. A number of outstanding materials are listed in Tables 1, 2 and 3 and referenced throughout the text. Table 1 includes sources of information on patient-centered care. Table 2 provides measurement and benchmarking resources and Table 3 has Quality improvement Tutorials and Toolkits. In addition to these resources, there are a number of models and tools that will be helpful for identifying desired outcomes for improved health care. For example, the "Clinical Value Compass" is a model that incorporates functional wellbeing, biological health, client satisfaction, and cost variables as potential outcomes that guide the development and evaluation of QI initiatives (TJC, 2007, p. 3).

Guided Inquiry

Review the most current National Quality Strategy priorities at http://ahrq.gov/workingfor quality/nqs.principles.htm (Table 2). Think about a common health problem encountered in your practice setting. Identify desired outcomes indicative of quality of care from the frame of reference of the patients and various members of the healthcare team.

Understanding the organizational context becomes an essential step in leading CQI. Systematic assessment of local context facilitates analysis of the problem, as well as identification of priorities for change. Research of high performing clinical microsystems has identified common themes associated with success that interact with one another, including leadership, staff, patients, performance, and information technology (Nelson, Batalden, Godfrey, & Eds., 2007) at http:/clinicalmicrosystem.org. The "Clinical Microsystem M3 Framework" provides a useful paradigm and many resources for assessing healthcare systems and identifying opportunities for improving care (Table 1)

(Nelson et al., 2011). One resource, the "Greenbook," details a comprehensive assessment of a clinical microsystem, including the "Purpose, Patient, Professionals, Processes, and Patterns" to lay the foundation for improvement at http:/clinicalmicrosystem.org.

Guided Inquiry

Locate the appropriate "Greenbook" for your practice setting and complete an assessment of the 5 Ps (purpose, patients, professionals, processes, and patterns). http://clinicalmicrosystem.org/materials/workbooks/

Does your workplace exhibit characteristics of a high-functioning microsystem?

The patient–provider dyad at the point of care represents the core or bull's-eye for enacting improvement in the care delivery process. Healthcare organizations and accrediting agencies have identified engagement of patients and families as partners in managing health as an essential component for improving the quality of health care; for example, the National Quality Strategy (AHRQ, 2011) and Partnership for Patients (USDHHS, 2011). Patient and family perspectives inform decisions and their compelling narratives incentivize meaningful changes across the spectrum of care. Intentionally involving the patient as a partner in care requires training and practice. As a member of the healthcare team, the nurse must be equipped to appropriately assess health literacy, to skillfully communicate options for healthcare management, and to identify strategies for shared decision making. Resources and tool kits for professionals and patients are available for guiding the shared decision-making process, as well as measuring patient-centered outcomes. (Web sites for several of these are provided in Table 1.) To promote meaningful improvements in healthcare quality, patients and families must be involved at multiple levels within the delivery system—extending beyond communicating personal care preferences to serving as advisors informing local as well as national policy.

Guided Inquiry

Falls either at home or in the hospital are often not witnessed. The Centers for Disease Control and Prevention (CDC) (2013) has created a toolkit that includes a patient-centered self-assessment tool, as well as guidelines for the health provider for addressing falls with patients. Explore the website and identify strategies for integrating shared decision making into your practice setting. http://www.cdc.gov/homeandrecreationalsafety/Falls/steadi/index.html

Table 1 Patient-centered Care Resources

Patient-centered Care	
Patient-centered Care Models as cited in Nelson, Batalden, Godfrey, & Lazar, 2011.	Anatomy of Clinical Microsystem 　http://clinicalmicrosystem.org/ Kano Model for Understanding Customer Satisfaction 　http://asq.org/learn-about-quality/qfd-quality-function-deployment/overview/kano-model.html Deming Model: Organizing as a System of Care Wagner's Chronic Care Model 　http://www.improvingchroniccare.org/ 　　index.php?p=The_Chronic_Care_Model&s=2 Lorig's Self-Management Model
Web Resources	Agency for Healthcare Research and Quality Engaging Patients and Families in the Quality and Safety of Hospital Care 　http://www.ahrq.gov/professionals/systems/hospital/ 　　engagingfamilies/index.html Center for Shared Decision Making 　http://patients.dartmouth-hitchcock.org/ 　　shared_decision_making.html ECRI Institute (National Patient Library & Home Care Resources) 　https://www.ecri.org/Patients/Pages/default.aspx The Healthcare and Patient Partnership Institute 　http://www.h2pi.org/ Informed Medical Decisions Foundation 　http://www.fimdm.org/ The Institute for Patient- and Family-Centered Care 　http://www.ipfcc.org/ National Patient Safety Foundation 　http://www.npsf.org/ Partnership for Patients 　http://partnershipforpatients.cms.gov/

Effectively involving patients in healthcare decisions is complicated by the complexity and unpredictability of health problems and outcomes. To understand quality and identify opportunities for improvement, it is essential to not only understand the complexity of the system, but also the complexity of the problems. Clinical problems are multi-faceted and often poorly defined, lacking a "one size fits all" solution. Efforts to standardize care, apply practice guidelines, and implement evidence-based practice (EBP) must make allowances for adapting to unique patient needs and contextual factors that are determinants of outcomes. Modifying the intervention to meet the unique needs of the local context is critical for successful planning and implementing of new initiatives. As a pivotal member of the healthcare team, the nurse care coordinator is well situated to leverage influence over the quality of clinical care—to lead meaningful changes in care quality.

BETTER PROFESSIONAL DEVELOPMENT

Professional Competency

The interrelationships between individuals and the surrounding context of care have implications for system enhancement, as well as for professional development. Professional development is the second pillar of Batalden and Davidoff's model. Nurses seek opportunities to improve quality on a daily basis through developing a reflective practice. Professional development, as a consequence of reflective practice and performance appraisal, requires the nurse to identify personal strengths and needs for further development based on an acute understanding of essential competencies. Participating in personal performance appraisals, formal peer review, clinical preceptorship, and informal mentoring requires understanding clinical competencies, critiquing care processes, and evaluating clinical outcomes. As depicted in the clinical microsystem framework, determination of professional needs must also incorporate competencies that address the unique needs of the clients served, as well as the challenges and resources within the context of care. The National Organization of Nurse Practitioner Faculties (2011) described the ability to apply skill in "peer review to promote a culture of excellence" that incorporates self-evaluation and monitoring of quality in own practice as a core competency to promote CQI.

Educational mandates espoused by national (IOM), professional (QSEN), and credentialing organizations [such as the American Nurses Credentialing Center (AACN) and National Organization of Nurse Practitioner Faculties (NONPF)] clearly articulate the core competencies required for healthcare team members to contribute to enhancing the safety of care and quality of outcomes. In the face of the knowledge explosion and the increasing complexity of health care, formal and informal networks have formed that offer communities of practice (COP) and learning for healthcare providers. Participating in a COP provides development of expertise and clinical decision-making while offering a platform for exploration of problems, sharing of successes, and encouragement. Research has shown that COPs are a key feature of successful implementation and sustaining quality initiatives (Aveling, Martin, Armstrong, Banerjee, & Dixon-Woods, 2012; Pronovost et al., 2010).

Exemplar—Communities of Practice (COP)

In early 2011, consumer attention and media coverage triggered increased attention to central line-associated bloodstream infection (CLABSI) rates in a 590-bed tertiary care hospital. Spurred by the moral and financial implications, an inter-disciplinary CLABSI workgroup was created and charged with minimizing CLABSI rates system-wide. The workgroup monitored CLABSI rates, reviewed current practice guidelines, made recommendations, and monitored compliance with practice guidelines. Those units that failed to meet the NDNQI® target rates were identified by CLABSI workgroup as the sites for QI projects. Participation of unit champions in the CLABSI workgroup provided a community of practice and learning that was essential to enhance knowledge, foster clinical expertise, and share successes and challenges.

Guided Inquiry

Identify a COP or networking group that is available to participate in or needed to enhance CQI efforts in your area of specialty.

Professional development depends upon thoughtful recognition of need and resources available, such as professional conferences, committees, professional networks, or self-directed tutorials (see Table 3 for examples). Membership in professional organizations and attendance at conferences provide strategic opportunities for professionals to network, gain clinical expertise, share experiences (formally or informally), and participate in leadership activities. A professional portfolio is a valuable tool for documenting accomplishments, identifying goals, and guiding professional development.

Guided Inquiry

Review the core *Quality* competencies from the Quality and Safety Education for Nurses (QSEN) initiative at http://qsen.org. Based on your professional work environment (reflect on the previous microsystem assessment), identify at least three areas where you have excelled. What personal attributes contributed to your success? What competencies need to be further developed?

The Academy of Healthcare Improvement (http://www.a4hi.org/home/) and IHI Open School (http://www.ihi.org/offerings/IHIOpenSchool/) provide various educational and networking opportunities. Based on the needs identified, review pertinent resources on each site and develop a strategy for professional development.

Change and Transformational Leadership

Cultivating a clear understanding of transformational leadership characteristics and principles for leading change are crucial components of professional development that will promote quality (IHI, 2013c). Informal and formal leadership opportunities and strategies are discussed in detail in Chapter 6. To be an effective leader in anticipating needs for change and in providing innovative coaching requires strong relationships with others, knowledge of personal influences, and adaptability. Understanding personal strengths and weaknesses facilitates identification of strategies to successfully collaborate with the project team and to engage staff in participating in a quality project and change practice on the unit. Appraisal of personal leadership traits through reflecting upon strengths and identifying strategies to enhance weaknesses establishes the foundation for cultivating skill as a change agent. Intentional exploration of personal traits enables the nurse to modify behaviors aimed at improving interactions with team members and key stakeholders. A variety of self-assessment tools are available to promote a non-biased analysis of personal styles.

Exemplar—Personality Assessment

The Myers-Briggs Type Indicator (MBTI®) is an inventory that assesses personality type, providing a framework used for personal and career development, leadership, teamwork, team building, workplace diversity, and business management. Review the descriptions of preferences described on the Myers-Briggs Foundation website and reflect on the potential barriers and facilitators to working with a team member with an "INFJ" personality type. (http://www.myersbriggs.org/)

Insights gained about personal characteristics enhance collaboration with others by promoting the ability to interpret responses, anticipate outcomes, and identify strategies for bettering communication. An essential component for improving healthcare quality is effective interprofessional collaboration. Health professions education has acknowledged the mandate to develop team skills and collaboration competencies (Interprofessional Education Collaborative Expert Panel, 2011). In addition, healthcare organizations have devoted resources (time and training) to strengthening team functioning to promote safety and quality. The Agency for Healthcare Research and Quality (AHRQ) in partnership with the Department of Defense have developed training materials and conferences that are widely distributed and shown to be effective in improving team skills (AHRQ, 2013.).

Thoughtful personal reflection paired with a clear framework for leading change provides direction and a strategy for interacting with other leaders in the healthcare arena and for overcoming resistance to change. Identifying strategies to promote change early in the process allows for planning to address resistance and sustain initiatives. Whether planning for individual or organizational change, foundational concepts emerge that characterize the change process. Successful programs strategically identify barriers and facilitators within the local context and build upon local success to scale up effective initiatives. For example, Kotter's stages of change provide a useful roadmap for creating a climate for change (building a sense of urgency, forming a team, and developing a shared vision), engaging and enabling the organization to embrace change (communicating buy-in, empowering broad-based action, and creating short-term wins), and implementing and sustaining change (maintain momentum and incorporate changes into culture) (Kotter International, 2012).

Guided Inquiry

Identify an opportunity to improve the quality of a healthcare process in your practice area (Reflect on national, organizational, or unit based priorities). Review the IHI "Knowledge Center: Forming a Team" (Institute for Healthcare Improvement, 2013b) and propose ideal team members to collaborate in improving care at: http://www.ihi.org/knowledge/Pages/HowtoImprove/ScienceofImprovementFormingtheTeam.aspx

Review templates for a meeting agenda at: http://clinicalmicrosystem.org/materials/worksheets/

Reflect on a recent team meeting and identify opportunities for improving the function and performance of the team.

Successful QI depends on effective leadership and strategic recruitment of team members. The team leader must identify key stakeholders (including patients, health team members, and administrators) to verify the full scope of the problem, to validate the processes involved, and to recruit proper organizational sponsors, champions, and local process owners. Creating a coalition and shared vision requires anticipating support needed to leverage resources necessary for implementing the project. Identifying barriers and facilitators, as well as addressing needs for workforce development early on and throughout a project, will promote future sustainability. Acquisition of resources needed to develop competencies for leading change efforts creates a foundation for integrating CQI into practice. To develop momentum for change, the team leader should consider involving those most resistant, those impacted by the change at the "sharp edge," namely the "customers" and the direct care providers, as well as those empowered to assure accountability and reward successes. Building an effective team and enlisting leadership support assures acquisition of needed resources and the power to promote success. Clarity of purpose, structure tailored to meet the unique needs of the group, well-organized meetings, and clear roles/responsibilities promote effective team work (Mitchell et al., 2012; The Dartmouth Institute, 2013). Agencies (such as the Institute for Healthcare Improvement and the Dartmouth Institute) that have formulated toolkits to guide QI methods incorporate resources for forming and organizing a team (Table 3) as integral to successfully implementing change.

Frameworks and Tools for Quality Improvement

Healthcare organizations have taken notice from other industries to identify frameworks for improving efficiency and enhancing quality. Conceptual frameworks and models for quality improvement offer strategies that support meaningful and systematic application of QI methods. Ideally, improvement is accomplished through rapid cycle changes that ultimately lead to widespread adoption. Incorporation of incremental change followed by analysis and revision, often referred to as PDSA (plan, do, study, act) is a feature of numerous models, including the Model for Improvement, Donabedian, Lean, and Six Sigma methods (see Table 3). The frameworks support ongoing reflection on practice and identification of opportunities for improvement that is continuously being evaluated and monitored. The Model for Improvement, for example, is the cornerstone for guiding healthcare improvement endorsed by the Institute for Healthcare Improvement (IHI, 2013b). The model presents a straight-forward template that addresses three main questions underlying continuous quality improvement: "What are we trying to accomplish; how will we know that a change is an improvement; what changes can we make that will result in improvement?" (IHI, 2013a, paragraph 1). Performance improvement teams utilizing Six Sigma methods focus on identifying and eliminating defects guided by the DMAIC approach (Define opportunities, Measure performance, Analyze opportunity, Improve performance, Control performance) (American Society for Quality, 2013).

Professional development in the realm of quality improvement becomes an essential component in achieving better healthcare outcomes. Engaging in a personal improvement project provides a framework for applying many of the improvement methods and tools, especially useful when learning the new concepts (Roberts & Sergesketter, 1993). Likewise, the experiential exercise allows one to gain greater insights into performance and work tendencies, as well as the implicit challenges to initiating and sustaining change. Training programs often integrate a personal improvement project as the capstone for the learning activity—regardless of the specific framework utilized. For example, applying the "Five S" concepts from Lean, a learner may seek opportunities to enhance efficiency in their own workspace by Sorting items in their office, determine a strategy to Set them in order, Simplify the filing system, Standardize the nomenclature, and Sustain the new work pattern. Incorporating the Model for Improvement, the plan will include measureable outcomes and a strategy for tracking and analyzing the data on a regular basis so that on-going modifications can be made.

Guided Inquiry

Reflect on a challenging clinical issue in your practice area. Identify opportunities for improvement by addressing the main questions posed by the Model for Improvement. (http://www.ihi.org/knowledge/Pages/HowtoImprove/default.aspx)

In response to comparisons with more rigorous research methods, scientists involved in QI work have developed numerous implementation models to increase the rigor and generalizability of QI work. Implementation science is research conducted to investigate how to best translate evidence into everyday practice (Duva, 2013). Models developed as a component of implementation science combine not only methods, but conceptual underpinnings that explain how interventions work, describe processes involved in implementation, guide analysis of outcomes, and sustain improvements. Concepts in models often capture principles associated with translating evidence into practice, change theory, social cognitive theory, self-regulation theory, systems theory, and team/group theory.

As depicted in one implementation model, the PARIHS Model, successful implementation of EBP is dependent upon the quality of the evidence, the quality of the context, and a person who can actively facilitate the evidence being translated into practice (Helfrich et al., 2010). Advanced practice nurses fulfill a pivotal role in providing leadership in effective implementation of evidence-based practice that is dependent upon the characteristics of leader as facilitator, the role in the organization, and personal style (Stetler, Damschroder, Helfrich, & Hagedorn, 2011). The process of translating evidence into practice includes identification of a clinical problem, review of the relevant literature, critical appraisal of the evidence, implementation of change in practice, and evaluation of practice change (Duva, 2013). Quality of evidence can be assessed using various approaches, such as the Joanna Briggs Institute's (2013) Model of Evidence-based Health Care FAME Scale (feasibility, appropriateness, meaningfulness, and effectiveness of interventions). Numerous other agencies provide guidance for evaluating evidence for quality improvement, such as the National Quality Forum (2011) and AHRQ (Owens et al., 2009).

Exemplar—Implementation Science Resources

The Veterans Healthcare Administration (VHA) has provided leadership and opportunities for the growth of implementation science providing resources and national expertise. Examples include: the VA Center for Implementation Practice and Research Support (CIPRS) (Veteran Adminstration's Health Services Research and Development Service, 2009); the "Enhancing Implementation Science" training program (Veteran Adminstration's Health Services Research and Development Service, 2013); and the VA *TAMMCS* guidebook to support members of the healthcare team to contribute to continuous improvements (Department of Veterans Affairs, 2011).

BETTER PATIENT AND SYSTEM OUTCOMES
Project Planning and Evaluation

To assure that changes implemented result in quality improvement, Batalden and Davidoff (2007) include a third pillar in their model, better patient and system outcomes. They describe essential knowledge elements to assist in planning and evaluating , including generalizable scientific evidence, characteristics of the particular context, strategies to promote change, and assessment of meaningful measures. Maintaining knowledge in one's practice area establishes the foundation for identification of gaps in practice, identification of problems, analysis of contributing factors, and creation of solutions. Determination of what to implement is accomplished by thoughtful review of the evidence for best practice; nurses' must be adept at locating, acquiring, and evaluating current evidence and translating it to the practice setting (TJC, 2007). A variety of strategies will assist the nurse in remaining appraised of the most up-to-date evidence in the select practice area, including participation in communities of learning, recurrent review of professional literature, and completion of continuing education. The National Guideline Clearinghouse, for example, publishes reviews of current evidence and recommends practice guidelines for a multitude of clinical problems. The IHI and the AHRQ publish innovative practice solutions that provide extensive evidence-based toolkits and resources for healthcare providers. In addition, specialty groups often create resource guides for healthcare providers, as well as for patients, to assist with the dissemination of the most current evidence.

Analyzing the scope of the problem involves identifying priorities and opportunities for improvement based upon the characteristics and needs of the local context in comparison to the relevant practice guidelines, benchmarks, or patient preferences. Fully understanding the problem and identifying needs for change requires adapting the

evidence based on an accurate appraisal of the clinical microsystem and systematic evaluation of variables impacting outcomes. Depending on the type of problem, there are a
variety of tools to assist in clarifying the multiple dimensions that define the problem,
such as a Pareto diagram, cause and effect (fishbone) diagram, or root cause analysis to
identify primary issues leading to a current problem and to identify an area for change
likely to have the greatest impact. Other strategies for identifying gaps, redundancies,
or inefficiencies include spaghetti diagrams or deployment, process, and value stream
mapping. Each diagrammatic representation allows the nurse to understand what the
current state is, to identify opportunities and vulnerabilities in a process, and to focus
improvement efforts. Generation of ideas for change can be stimulated by applying overarching change concepts, such as eliminating, reordering, replacing, or combining steps
to name a few (TJC, 2007).

Exemplar—Targets for Improvement

The Joint Commission (2007) has identified 14 strategies for identifying
targets for improvement in clinical care:

1. Talk to insiders; ask the staff
2. Engage the beneficiaries of clinical care—ask patients, their families, and other stakeholders
3. See what others have done—explore the literature
4. Read about what works—check out case study reports
5. Look at what others know about local practice—from the outside
   looking in
6. Treasure the defects—if it's broken, fix it
7. Understand "competitors"
8. Check out the customer survey results
9. Understand the current process
10. Walk in their shoes—play the role
11. Review the internal data
12. Identify the sink hole of temporary help
13. Eliminate waste
14. Probe the process more deeply—use change concepts

The success of improvement work depends on the formation of high functioning
teams. Teams will vary in composition and size depending upon the needs of the project.
A well-rounded team includes representation of key stakeholders, such as clinical leaders,
technical experts, day-to-day leaders, project sponsor, or patients. Fully understanding
the nature of the problem and processes involved equips the team to generate multiple

options for change focused on achieving the aims. The project team may seek insights from those who work in the system, brainstorm change concepts or other creative thinking techniques, or borrow from the experience of others who have successfully improved a similar situation (IHI, 2013b). Effective group work strategies will assist in promoting open exchange of ideas and fluidity in building consensus when determining priorities, establishing realistic aims, and creating feasible interventions. Open communication, clearly understood member roles, and shared responsibility leads to a high functioning team. Building consensus can be facilitated in numerous ways, such as brainstorming and multi-voting. Intentional team building activities that promote the establishment of relationships and a shared vision paired with effective leadership form the foundation for initiating change. Useful strategies and programs have been developed to promote effective team skills (e.g., TeamSTEPPS and the list of selected references at the end of the chapter).

Successful implementation of a program to improve outcomes requires a clear plan for implementation, communication, and training (Duva, 2013). The implementation plan addresses what is being implemented, by whom, when, and how success will be evaluated. Once an intervention is identified, an action plan that provides a timeline with key milestones will assist in setting priorities and managing time. A workflow diagram or Gantt chart assists in mapping out and organizing key components of a project. Planning should also outline a proposed budget that identifies all resources anticipated for implementation. The communication plan, with project team members and key stakeholders, identifies who needs to know about the change, as well as how and when communications should be distributed. Planning for adequate team training regarding the implementation and evaluation methods will promote efficiency, reliability and validity of work, and sustainability of the initiative. There are many educational resources and tools to guide project development, implementation, and evaluation (AHRQ, 2008; DVA, 2011; Harvard Business Essentials, 2004; TJC, 2007; Ogrinfc et al., 2012). (For additional resources see Table 3 and the list of selected references at the end of the chapter.)

Assessment of Meaningful Quality Measures

Performance and outcome measures defined by accreditation, reimbursement, and professional organizations motivate policy makers and healthcare leaders to initiate or support QI work, as well as recognize excellence. Metrics can be used to identify population needs, evaluate individual patient outcomes, and assess quality of care provided.

Utilizing an implementation framework guides selection of metrics to evaluate the effectiveness of a QI initiative. The IHI Model for Improvement, for example, links aims, measures, and change concepts with rapid cycle change (IHI, 2012). Clearly defined aims allow determination of whether a planned change made a difference in outcomes. The aim should define the specific population of patients that will be affected by the change (TJC, 2007). An aim is characterized by objectives that include criteria that are specific, measurable, achievable, realistic, and have a time frame (SMART) (Ogrinc et al., 2012). SMART objectives allow the project team to identify key measures that will be utilized to assess the baseline and to evaluate the outcomes.

Clearly defined measures allow not only for the determination of whether a planned change made a difference in outcomes, but also the evaluation of the fidelity of the implementation (process measure), and assessment for any unintended effects (balancing measure). Evaluation of interventions and outcomes occurs throughout and at the conclusion of the designated time frame established for the implementation. If the outcomes are not achieved, all aspects of the planning need to be reviewed, including the evidence for the solution, contextual factors, and processes involved. With financial and personnel resources becoming scarcer, well-defined project aims and measures assist in leveraging results to justify allocation of resources.

Significant learning can result from thoughtful reflection on the results of a change project, and can lead to ideas for revision and strategies for sustaining the change and scaling up the initiative to have a greater reach. When applied to QI work, learning from defects becomes integral to the change process. For example, audit results shared with those at the point of care provide "just in time" feedback that promotes professional efficacy, buy-in, and motivation to sustain improvement efforts (Pronovost, Berenholtz, & Needham, 2008; Pronovost et al., 2010). The ability to learn from defects or errors has been described as an essential ingredient for cultivating a culture of safety within an organization (IHI, 2008). A variety of useful toolkits have been created as guides for planning, implementing, and evaluating QI projects.

Many healthcare organizations utilize internal, as well as external, databases to guide decision-making to plan and evaluate quality initiatives. It is essential for healthcare providers to understand how to effectively use key metrics. For example, how to identify,

Case In Point

In reviewing the most up-to-date evidence to guide policy recommendations for the Falls Prevention Program, the sub-committee sought guidance from a multitude of sources. Compare and contrast resources available at the NGC, AHRQ, IHI, HRSA, and the VA NCPS websites. (Table 3)

access, and analyze national and local databases as the baseline for planning and evaluating. A benchmark serves as a reference point for establishing aims and is an important point of reference to answer the question of whether an improvement or change made a difference. Sometimes the benchmark consists solely of baseline measures to compare one microsystem to itself over time, whereas national benchmark measures are available for other outcomes, such as readmission rates. Selecting the proper target and comparison group is also important to assure validity of conclusions and to promote efforts to sustain or scale up interventions. (See Table 2 for benchmarking and measurement databases.)

Guided Inquiry

Visit the CMS website "Hospital Compare" at http://medicare.gov/hospitalcompare/?AspxAutoDetectCookieSupport=1.

   Compare quality of care for three hospitals in your market area and identify QI priorities.

Development of specific measures to monitor processes and outcomes with a well-articulated system for data collection provides data useful for analysis and determining revisions. Critical analysis of the aims and measures reveals the types of data that will be needed. Some standardized criteria for performance and outcome measures have been defined: participants must properly collect, track, and interpret appropriate data, such as data reported to NDNQI® on falls. The data collection plan must specify not only what data to collect, but also how, by whom, and how frequently. The plan must be communicated clearly to team members, specify training needs, and address strategies to avoid negative impact on workflow and measure fatigue. The data collection process also serves as an opportunity to provide "just in time" feedback to participants, especially when defects are identified. Examples of data collection tools include surveys, checklists, or tally sheets utilizing a variety of data collection methods, such as chart review, interview, or observation. Standardized instruments have been developed enhancing the validity and reliability of the results. Information technology plays a pivotal role in facilitating QI work, incorporating methods for data collection, data management, and data analysis. A multitude of resources provide sample instruments and templates to guide the development of appropriate measures and reliable data collection.

With the growing attention to healthcare improvement, many healthcare organizations have resources and an infrastructure in place to support data collection and reporting, such as TheraDoc™ Clinical Surveillance System (2012). To assist in developing a data management plan, the nurse must be knowledgeable about available databases and

Table 2 Benchmarking and Measurement Resources

CMS Partnership for Patients	http://partnershipforpatients.cms.gov/
Dartmouth Atlas Project – Efficiency and Effectiveness of the Health Care System	http://www.dartmouthatlas.org/
Hospital Compare	http://medicare.gov/ hospitalcompare/?AspxAutoDetectCookieSupport=1
Institute for Improvement: Improvement Map	http://www.ihi.org/offerings/Initiatives/ Improvemaphospitals/Pages/default.aspx?TabId=2
The Joint Commission: ORYX measures	http://www.jointcommission.org/ www.qualitycheck.org
National Committee for Quality Assurance Health: Effectiveness Data and Information Set	http://www.ncqa.org/HomePage.aspx
National Database of Nursing Quality Indicators® (NDNQI®)	https://www.nursingquality.org/default.aspx
National Healthcare Safety Network (NHSN)	http://www.cdc.gov/nhsn/
National Quality Forum (NQF)	http://www.qualityforum.org/Home.aspx
National Quality Strategy	http://www.ahrq.gov/workingforquality/nqs/principles. htm
Working for Quality: National Quality Strategy	http://www.ahrq.gov/workingforquality/index.html

resources in their local system. Understanding of the type of data will enable the most accurate and compelling representation and analysis of the data. For example, many measures are tracked over time and, when represented as a simple run chart, the results may be misinterpreted. Understanding statistical process control charts (SPC) allows for more in-depth and meaningful interpretation of results. Gaining competency in utilizing and interpreting healthcare data requires training and support. Review the resources listed in Table 3 and the American Society for Quality's "Learn About Quality" (ASQ, 2013).

Communication of Results

Lastly, the project plan describes the strategies for communicating results to the key stakeholders. Formative summaries are helpful to sustain engagement for those most affected by the change and to celebrate key milestone and success (all useful strategies for successfully changing processes). Formal and informal summaries provide the foundation for scaling up successful programs. Key messages to include in an executive summary include description of the program methods, outcomes, cost implications (value

Table 3 QI Tutorials and Toolkits

Quality Improvement Tutorials and Toolkits	
Academy for Healthcare Improvement-Educational Resources	http://www.a4hi.org/home/
Aligning Forces for Quality—Collaboratives, Tools, and Resources	http://forces4quality.org/
AHRQ Quality Toolkits	http://www.ahrq.gov/qual/qitoolkit
	http://www.ahrq.gov/professionals/systems/hospital/qitoolkit/qiroadmap.html
HRSA Quality Toolkit	http://www.hrsa.gov/quality/toolbox/index.html
Institute for Healthcare Improvement IHI Open School- Tutorials	http://www.ihi.org/offerings/IHIOpenSchool/overview/Pages/default.aspx
Institute for Healthcare Improvement	http://www.ihi.org/knowledge/Pages/default.aspx
Interprofessional Education Collaborative	http://www.aacn.nche.edu/education-resources/ipecreport.pdf
QSEN (Quality and Safety Education for Nurses)	http://qsen.org/
Six Sigma—Tutorials and Tools	http://sixsigmatutorial.com/
	www.dmaictools.com
TeamSTEPPS—Team Training	http://teamstepps.ahrq.gov/
Transforming Care At Bedside	http://www.ihi.org/offerings/Initiatives/PastStrategicInitiatives/TCAB/Pages/default.aspx
Quality Improvement Resources	
American Society for Quality (ASQ)	http://asq.org/knowledge-center/index.html
AHRQ: Grading the Strength of Evidence	http://www.effectivehealthcare.ahrq.gov
AHRQ Morbidity & Mortality Cases	http://www.webmm.ahrq.gov
Clinical Microsystems	http://clinicalmicrosystem.org/materials/worksheets/
Institute of Medicine	http://www.iom.edu/
Institute for Clinical Systems Improvement (ICSI)	https://www.icsi.org/
Institute for Safe Medication Practices	http://ismp.org/
Joanna Briggs Institute Model of Evidence-based Health Care	www.joannabriggs.edu.au
National Center for Nursing Quality® (NCNQ®)	http://www.nursingworld.org/MainMenuCategories/ThePracticeofProfessionalNursing/PatientSafetyQuality
National Guideline Clearinghouse	http://www.guideline.gov/
Robert Wood Johnson Foundation	http://www.rwjf.org/en/about-rwjf/program-areas.html
SQUIRE- Standards for Quality Improvement Reporting Excellence	http://squire-statement.org/
TheraDocTM Clinical Surveillance System	http://www.theradoc.com/solutions/quality-improvement/
VA National Center for Patient Safety	http://www.patientsafety.gov/

added estimations or return on investment), and recommendations. Sharing outcomes to external stakeholders by creating a story board, presenting findings at a conference, or publishing in a professional journal contribute to the growing body of knowledge and communities of learning focused on improving healthcare outcomes. Resources included in Table 3 include guidelines for calculating return on investment (e.g., ASQ) and publication (SQUIRE).

Nurses involved in CQI need to be knowledgeable about what metrics are reported nationally and how the reports are reflective of nursing practice. The American Nurses Association has provided exceptional leadership in acknowledging the essential role nurses serve in achieving quality patient outcomes and in providing an infrastructure (NDNQI®) for data reporting (ANA, 2013). Organizations seeking certification by the Magnet Recognition Program® often have robust processes for monitoring and reporting quality metrics. The formation of nation-wide databases of performance and outcome measures has allowed organizations to make meaningful comparisons with similar organizations, to identify benchmarks, and to set goals for continuous improvement. Assessing performance using dashboards focused on key quality indicators allows leaders to identify gaps and opportunities, as well as track change over time. The IHI Improvement Map (2013a) is an example of a dashboard, a web-based interactive tool to guide and document improvements (safety, transitions, cost) particularly addressing the nine core focus areas identified by Partnership for Patients (CMS, n.d.). Each map includes a framework for improvement processes that details elements of the process, outcome measures, service lines/critical functions, implications (patient/family, standards/policy, financial, prerequisites) and resources. (See Tables 1 and 2.)

SUMMARY OF NURSING'S QI ROLE

Learning and practicing QI within different healthcare settings has highlighted guiding principles that are foundational for promoting change. First, as depicted in the Pillars of QI Model, quality is everyone's job (Batalden & Davidoff, 2007). Developing competencies in quality improvement begins with cultivating a personal commitment to continually seek opportunities for improving within one's personal life as well as professional life. Second is the need to establish effective respectful relationships with others. A practice of reflection and introspection paired with open regard for contributions of all involved in a situation promotes a culture of collaboration and foundation for change. Including the voice and values of the patient as a customer and key stakeholder is essential for identifying meaningful outcomes and feasible interventions. Third, to be effective, change agents must empower decision making at the point of patient contact and service. Effective

---

Case In Point

CLABSI calculator is one example of a tool to estimate cost savings. In one year, a cardiovascular thoracic ICU (an 18-bed unit) recorded eight CLABSIs. Based on "The CLASBI Opportunity Estimator" (JHQSRG, 2005–2009) the unit and hospital likely incurred a cost of one avoidable death, $320,000–$368,563.65 when adjusted for inflation and 64 unnecessary days in the ICU. By reducing the CLABSI rate approximately 75%, the unit and organization potentially saved $240,000/year based on previous rates.

In coordinating care for patient populations, healthcare providers often monitor performance and outcomes across a larger health system. Healthcare systems also participate in voluntary and mandatory reporting of performance and outcome measures that are utilized for accreditation (TJC, NHSN), credentialing (ANCC), and reimbursement (CMS).

---

change agents recognize relationships within and between systems and strive to engage those most affected by change as partners in identifying solutions and sustaining change. Fourth, QI work must be process and data driven. A systematic approach to QI rooted within a conceptual framework allows small incremental change, as well as broadscale organizational change. Lastly, leadership sets the tone for quality and safety for a learning organization.

A "learning organization" provides leadership support, resources, and an infrastructure to promote change and quality as an integrated aspect of the work of a healthcare team. Members of an organization need to understand the local culture and drivers (priorities for action) to effectively promote change within a given context. A community of practice and learning promotes professional development—an invaluable opportunity for individuals to share experiences and problems, brainstorm possible solutions, build expertise, and gain momentum in leading and sustaining change.

Sometimes QI is characterized as changing system structures and processes using nice, concrete tools and skills such as PDSA cycles, the Model of Improvement, Lean, Six Sigma, flow maps, fishbone diagrams, control charts, etc. While those are important, the best project plan in the world will have a less than ideal chance of success if the right mix of people is not on board, if necessary resources are not identified and made available for the project, and if local context, organizational culture, and will are not taken into account and utilized. Ongoing engagement, education, execution, and evaluation (4E's Model) are required for seeking opportunities to improve care and to sustain/build upon successes (Pronovost, Berenholtz, & Needham, 2008).

Case In Point

As a clinical nurse leader in a large integrated health system, you have been asked to lead a new interprofessional committee on preventing falls and fall-related injury. As a relative newcomer, what do you need to understand about the context or system? What are possible drivers for the appointment of this committee?

- Leadership messages
- Organizational and unit level processes related to falls
- Resources devoted to preventing falls
- Variety of clinical care contexts and services provided
- Characteristics of patient population
- Characteristics of healthcare team
- System vulnerabilities and opportunities for improving care
- Sense of urgency or motivation for decision to create committee

See sample toolkit: *Preventing Falls in Hospitals—A Toolkit for Improving Quality of Care* at http://www.ahrq.gov/professionals/systems/long-term-care/resources/injuries/fallpxtoolkit/index.html

CONCLUSION

An understanding of quality improvement models and tools is essential for active and meaningful participation in health reform and advancing care coordination practice. The systems orientation to quality improvement presented in this chapter provides an important foundation for realizing quality outcomes and the benefits of care coordination. We cannot achieve better outcomes without simultaneous improvements in system performance and professional development. These goals require that all health professionals engage in continuous quality improvement and systematically apply its principles and tools in all areas of practice. This is especially true for care coordination practices that rely on exquisite system integration and skilled professionals able to effectively navigate at the intersections of a complex health system. It is not surprising that care coordination has emerged as a priority for improving quality and safety. Achieving its intended outcomes requires embedding care coordination in rigorous and continuous improvement.

REFERENCES

Agency for Healthcare Research and Quality (AHRQ). (2013). TeamSTEPPS: National implementation. Retrieved from http://teamstepps.ahrq.gov/

Agency for Healthcare Research and Quality (AHRQ). (2011). Working for quality: The national quality strategy.

Agency for Healthcare Research and Quality (AHRQ). (n.d.). Principles for the National Quality Strategy (NQS). Retreived from http://www.ahrq.gov/workingforquality/nqs/principles.htm

American Nurses Association (ANA). (2013). NDNQI home page. Retrieved from http://www.nursingquality.org/

Aveling, E. L, Martin, G., Armstrong, N., Banerjee, J., & Dixon-Woods, M. (2012). Quality improvement through clinical communities: Eight lessons for practice. *Journal of Health Organization and Management, 26*(2), 158–174.

Batalden, P. B., & Davidoff, F. (2007). What is "quality improvement" and how can it transform healthcare? *Quality and Safety in Health Care, 16*(1), 2–3. doi: 10.1136/qshc.2006.022046

Center for Medicare and Medicaid Services (CMS) (n.d.) Partnership for Patients. Retrieved from http://partnershipforpatients.cms.gov/

Dartmouth Institute. (2013). Clinical microsystems: Workbooks. Retrieved from http://clinicalmicrosystem.org/materials/workbooks/

Department of Veterans Affairs (DVA). (2011). *VA TAMMCS: Improvement framework guidebook.* Washington, DC: Author.

Duva, Ingrid. (2013). *What is implementation science.* Presentation. Nell Hodgson Woodruff School of Nursing, Emory University. Atlanta, GA.

Helfrich, C. D., Damschroder, L. J., Hagedorn, H. J., Daggett, G. S., Sahay, A., Ritchie, M.,… Stetler, C. B. (2010). A critical synthesis of literature on the promoting action on research implementation in health services (PARIHS) framework. *Implement Sci, 5*, 82. doi: 10.1186/1748-5908-5-82

Institute for Healthcare Improvement (IHI). (2008). *Prevent central line infections how to guide.* Cambridge, MA: Author.

Institute for Healthcare Improvement (IHI). (2012). How to Improve. Retrieved from http://www.ihi.org/knowledge/Pages/HowtoImprove/default.aspx

Institute for Healthcare Improvement (IHI). (2013a). On Demand: An introduction to the Model for Improvement. Retrieved from http://www.ihi.org/offerings/virtualprograms/ondemand/improvementmodelintro/Pages/default.aspx

Institute for Healthcare Improvement (IHI). (2013b). Knowledge center: How to improve. Retrieved from http://www.ihi.org/knowledge/Pages/HowtoImprove/default.aspx

Institute for Healthcare Improvement (IHI). (2013c). Transforming care at the bedside. Retrieved from http://www.ihi.org/offerings/Initiatives/PastStrategicInitiatives/TCAB/Pages/default.aspx

Interprofessional Education Collaborative Expert Panel. (2011). *Core competencies for interprofessional collaborative practice*: Report of an expert panel. Washington, DC: Author.

Joanna Briggs Institute. (2013). Levels of evidence: FAME. Retrieved from http://www.joannabriggs.edu.au/Levels%20of%20Evidence%20%20FAME

John Hopkins Hospital Quality and Safety Research Group (JHQSRG), (2005–2009). Stop BSI: CLABSI opportunity estimator. Retrieved from http://www.hopkinsmedicine.org/quality_safety_research_group/our_projects/stop_bsi/toolkits_resources/clabsi_estimator.html

The Joint Commission. (TJC). (2007). *Practice-based learning and improvement: A clinical improvement action guide* (2nd ed.). E. C. Nelson, P. B. Batalden, & J. S. Lazar (Eds.). Oak Brook, IL: Joint Commission Resources.

Kotter International. (2012). The 8-step process for leading change. Retrieved from http://www.kotterinternational.com/our-principles/changesteps/changesteps

Mitchell, P. H. , Wynia, M., Golden, R. , McNellis, B. , Okun, S., Webb, C.E., ... Von Kohorn, I. (2012). *Core principles and values of effective team-based health care.* Retrieved from www.iom.edu/tbc

National Organization of Nurse Practitioner Faculties. (2011). Competencies for nurse practitioners. Retrieved from http://www.nonpf.com/

National Quality Forum (NQF). (2011). Guidance for evaluating the evidence related to the focus of quality measurement and importance to measure and report. Retrieved from http://www.qualityforum.org/Publications/2011/01/Evidence_Task_Force.aspx

Nelson, E. C., Batalden, P. B., Godfrey, M. M., & Eds. (2007). *Quality by design: a clinical microsystems approach.* San Francisco, CA: Jossey-Bass.

Ogrinc, G. S., Headrick, L. A., Moore, S. M., Barton, A. J., Dolansky, M. A., & Madigosky, W. S. (2012). *Fundamentals of health care improvement: A guide to improving your patient's care* (2nd ed.). Oakbrook, IL: The Joint Commission & Institute for Healthcare Improvement.

Owens, D. K., Lohr, K. N., Atkins, D., Treadwell, J. R., Reston, J. T., Bass, E. B., ... Helfand, M. (2009). Grading the strength of a body of evidence when comparing medical interventions. In *Agency for healthcare research and quality. Methods guide for comparative effectiveness reviews.* Rockville, MD: Agency for Healthcare Research and Quality. Retrieved from http://www.effectivehealthcare.ahrq.gov/index.cfm/search-for-guides-reviews-and-reports/?pageaction=displayproduct&productid=328.

Pronovost, P. J., Goeschel, C. A., Colantuoni, E., Watson, S. R., Lubomski, L. H., Berenholtz, S. M., & Needham, D. (2010). Sustaining reductions in catheter related bloodstream infections in Michigan intensive care units: Observational study. *British Medical Journal.* doi: 10.1136/bmj.c309

Pronovost, P. J., Berenholtz, S. M., & Needham, D. M. (2008). Translating evidence into practice: A model for large scale knowledge translation. *BMJ, 337.* doi: 10.1136/bmj.a1714

Stetler, C. B., Damschroder, L. J., Helfrich, C. D., & Hagedorn, H. J. (2011). A Guide for applying a revised version of the PARIHS framework for implementation. *Implement Science, 6,* 99. doi: 10.1186/1748-5908-6-99

TheraDoc Inc. (2012). TheraDoc solutions: Quality improvement. Retrieved from http://www.theradoc.com/solutions/quality-improvement/

U.S. Department of Health & Human Services. (2011). Partnership for patients: Better care, lower costs. Retrieved from http://www.healthcare.gov/news/factsheets/2011/04/partnership04122011a.html

Veteran Adminstration's Health Services Research and Development Service. (2009). QUERI implementation guide. Retrieved from http://www.queri.research.va.gov/implementation/

Veteran Adminstration's Health Services Research and Development Service. (2013). QUERI: meetings – enhancing implementation science in VA. Retrieved from http://www.queri.research.va.gov/meetings/

Selected References on Quality

Agency for Healthcare Research and Quality. (2008). *Patient safety and quality: An evidence-based handbook for nurses.* Rockville, MD: Author. http://www.ahrq.gov/professionals/clinicians-providers/resources/nursing/resources/nurseshdbk/index.html

Agency for Healthcare Research and Quality. (2005). *A toolkit for redesign in health care: Final report.* Rockville, MD: Author. http://www.ahrq.gov/professionals/quality-patient-safety/patient-safety-resources/resources/toolkit/index.html

Amer, K.S. (2013). *Quality and safety for transformational nursing: Core competencies.* Upper Saddle River, NJ: Pearson.

Brassard, M., & Ritter, D. (1994). *Memory jogger II.* Methuen, MA: GOAL/QPC.

Brassard, M. (1995). *The team memory jogger.* Methuen, MA: GOAL/QPC.

Carey, R. G., & Stake, L.V. (2003). *Improving healthcare with control charts: Basic and advanced SPC methods and case studies.* Milwaukee, WI: ASQ Quality Press.

George, M., Maxey, J., Rowlands, D., & Upton, M. (2005). *The Lean Six Sigma pocket toolbook: A quick reference guide to 70 tools for improving quality and speed.* New York: McGraw Hill.

Griener, A. C., & Knebel, E. (2003). *Health professions education: A bridge to quality.* Washington, DC: National Academy Press.

Hadfield, D., Holmes, S., Kozlowski, S., & Sperl, T. (2009). *The Lean healthcare pocket guide: Tools for the elimination of waste in hospitals, clinics, and other healthcare facilities.* Chelsea, MI: MCS Media, Inc.

Harvard Business Essentials. (2004). *Managing projects large and small: The fundamental skills for delivering on budget and on time.* Boston: Harvard Business School Press.

Institute of Medicine. (2001). *Crossing the quality chasm: A new health system for the 21st century.* Washington, DC: National Academy Press.

Joint Commission on Accreditation of Healthcare Organizations. (1996). *Pocket guide to using performance improvement tools.* Oakbrook Terrace, IL: Joint Commission on Accreditation of HealthCare Organizations.

Kohn, L. T., Corrigan, J. M., & Donaldson, M. S. (1999). *To err is human: Building a safer health system.* Washington, DC: National Academy Press.

Langley, G., Nolan, K., Nolan, T., Norman, C., & Provost, L. (1996). *The improvement guide: A practical approach to enhancing organizational performance.* San Francisco, CA: Jossey-Bass.

Nelson, E.C., Batalden, P.B., & Lazar, J.S., Eds. (2007). *Practice-Based learning and improvement: A clinical improvement action guide (2nd Edition).* Oakbrook Terrace, IL: Joint Commission on Accreditation of HealthCare Organizations.

Nelson, E., Batalden, P., & Godfrey M. (2007). *Quality by design: A clinical microsystems approach.* San Francisco, CA: Jossey-Bass.

Nelson, E., Batalden, P., Godfrey, M., & Lazar, J.S. (2011). *Value by design: Developing clinical microsystems to achieve organizational excellence.* San Francisco, CA: Josse-Bass.

Ogrinc, G. S., Headrick, L. A., Moore, S. M., Barton, A. J., Dolansky, M. A., & Madigosky, W. S. (2012). *Fundamentals of health care improvement.* Oakbrook Terrace, IL: The Joint Commission and the Institute for Healthcare Improvement.

Roberts, H., & Sergesketter, B. (1993). *Quality is personal: A foundation for total quality management.* New York: The Free Press.

Rutherford P., Phillips, J., Coughlan, P., Lee, B., Moen, R., Peck, C., & Taylor, J. (2008) *Transforming care at the bedside how-to guide: Engaging front-line staff in innovation and quality improvement.* Cambridge, MA: Institute for Healthcare Improvement. Available at www.IHI.org.

Sherwood, G., & Barnsteiner, J. (2012). *Quality and safety in nursing: A competency approach to improving outcomes.* Hoboken, NJ: Wiley-Blackwell.

Scholtes, P. R., Joiner, B. L., & Streibel, B. J. (2003). *The team handbook: How to use teams to improve quality* (3rd ed.). Madison, WI: Oriel Incorporated.

Section 2

Care Coordination: Practice and Leadership

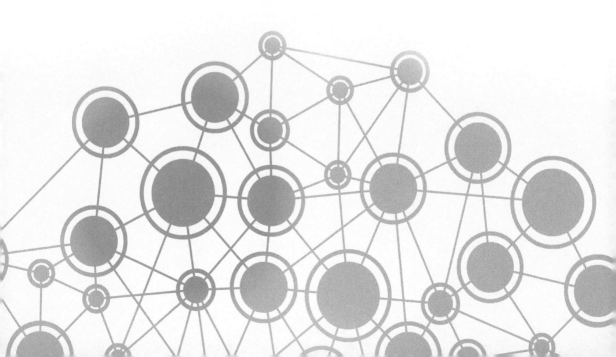

Chapter 4

Effective Care Coordination Models

Cheryl Schraeder, PhD, RN, FAAN and Paul Shelton, EdD

Changing demographics, behaviors, and lifestyles have had a dramatic impact on public health and disease characteristics of the U.S. population. These changes, coupled with increased longevity, have resulted in individuals living with illnesses that are chronic, complex to manage, and very expensive to treat. The increasing incidence of chronic illness among Americans poses major challenges to a healthcare system that currently consumes 17% of the nation's gross domestic product (Schimpff, 2012), and that is projected to increase to 20% by the end of this decade (Keehan et al., 2011). These rising healthcare costs are unsustainable and are having major fiscal impacts on state governments, the federal Medicare and Medicaid programs, and out-of-pocket expenses incurred by individuals.

The percentage of adults with one or more chronic conditions is a major driving force behind the nation's accelerating healthcare costs (Reuben, 2007). Estimations are that 25% of all Americans are diagnosed with multiple chronic conditions (MCC), and 75% aged 65 years and older have MCC (Ward & Schiller, 2013; Tinetti, Fried, & Boyd, 2012). Individuals with MCC are the major consumers of healthcare services and account for over 66% of total healthcare spending (Anderson, 2010). As the number of chronic conditions affecting an individual increase, so do consequences such as an increase in preventable hospital admissions, adverse drug events/medication errors, duplication of care, conflicting medical advice, poor functional status, and unnecessary pain and suffering (Parekh & Barton, 2010).

Not surprisingly, our current healthcare system, with an emphasis on acute care and managing individual diseases, is unable to provide high quality care for these individuals. The Institute of Medicine (IOM) has called for fundamental changes in how all health care is delivered, especially chronic illness care that is fragmented and dysfunctional (IOM, 2001). Change has been slow in coming, primarily due to an outdated fee-for-service financial system that rewards duplication of services and unnecessary care (Parekh & Barton, 2010), exceptionally slow adoption of information technology, and a general lack of incentives to change the way care is delivered (Reuben, 2007).

Although the future of healthcare reform is still uncertain, recent legislation (Affordable Care Act, American Recovery and Reinvestment Act, and Health Information Technology for Economic and Clinical Health Act) provides the federal government with mechanisms to realign incentives and payments to improve service delivery (Blumenthal, 2012). Significant areas the legislation addresses include failures in care delivery, the lack of widespread adoption of best care processes, and failures of care coordination when chronically ill patients fall through the cracks of a fragmented care delivery system (Berwick & Hackbarth, 2012). Coordinated care programs, such as patient-centered medical homes (PCMHs) and accountable care organizations (ACOs), have been incorporated into health reform legislation as promising approaches to strengthen primary care in an effort to improve quality and reduce costs.

Over the past two decades, a number of researchers have developed and tested models to improve the care for persons with chronic illnesses, primarily older adults insured through Medicare and Medicaid. These programs are broadly based on the chronic care model (Coleman, Austin, Brach, & Wagner, 2009), and involve physicians, registered nurses (RNs), and other professionals working in collaborative teams with patients and their caregivers to implement evidence-based best practices and provide comprehensive coordinated care. The primary goals of these programs are to reduce avoidable hospital admissions and to improve patients' quality of life and satisfaction with care.

Achieving improvements in the care for MCC individuals has been difficult. Understanding how to care for these individuals is one of the most important challenges facing the healthcare industry (Vogeli et al., 2007). Published results from these clinical trials and demonstrations have provided evidence for improved care processes, quality of life, and satisfaction with care, as well as limited success in reduced use and cost of health services. Since the programs varied in target patient populations, implementation settings, and the number of intervention components incorporated into each model, more vigorous evaluation studies are required to determine what constitutes best chronic illness care (Bettger et al., 2012; de Bruin et al., 2012; Hansen, Young, Hinami, Leung, & Williams, 2011). However, despite limited success, the results suggest that certain model components are integral to care management, and have the potential to be cost effective in efforts to manage adults with MCC. In addition, the results indicate that when RNs are an integral part of direct care through the management of the interdisciplinary team, programs have the best opportunity to improve clinical outcomes and reduce expenditures.

This chapter will review over 20 years of research and practice in care coordination that can be used as a resource for the improvement of chronic care delivery. Topics covered include a brief review of the care coordination evidence, the components and practices of effective care coordination, the roles that RNs perform in effective care coordination, skills that RNs will need to be key players in the future of a transformed healthcare delivery system, and steps to take in the future for effective care coordination to become a reality.

THE CARE COORDINATION EVIDENCE-BASE

A growing body of literature suggests effective care coordination interventions hold promise to improve care delivery and reduce overall costs for adults with MCC, especially if the most effective care coordination components can be identified and implemented (Brown, 2009). Effectiveness requires rigorous evidence from either a randomized controlled trial or a quasi-experimental comparison group design, and improved patient outcomes *with* a reduction in healthcare expenditures through reduced hospitalizations. Improved clinical indicators and patient satisfaction alone are not considered effective evidence. Effective care coordination and care management interventions fall into two general categories: transitional care and coordinated care. Although both approaches have common elements, they differ on when and where the intervention begins, how it is staffed, and how long it lasts.

Transitional Care

Promising transitional care interventions include the Transitional Care Model (TCM), Care Transitions Intervention (CTI), Project Re-Engineered Discharge (RED), and Enhanced Discharge Planning Program (EDPP). Although each intervention model is different, the interventions:

- Target and engage patients with chronic illnesses while hospitalized to prepare them for a smooth transition home;
- Follow patients intensively for a short period of time, usually from one to 12 weeks post-discharge;
- Teach/coach patients about their medications, self-care, and symptom recognition and management; and
- Remind, encourage, and assist patients to attend follow-up appointments with their primary care provider (PCP).

The TCM, developed by Naylor and colleagues (2012), utilizes a multidisciplinary team to provide evidence-based protocols, led by an advanced practice transitional care nurse (TCN). TCNs follow patients who have complex chronic conditions for 12 weeks after the index hospitalization. TCM achieved lower re-hospitalization rates and lower mean total costs after 12 months for intervention patients (Naylor et al., 1999; Naylor et al., 2004). The TCI, developed by Coleman and colleagues (2004), is a self-management model. A transition coach, who can be an advanced practice registered nurse, registered nurse, social worker, or occupational therapist, follows patients post-discharge for one month, provides them with tools to promote communication among their specialty care providers, and encourages them to take a more active role in their care. Intervention patients had lower re-admission rates at 30 and 90 days and lower average hospital costs at 180 days (Coleman et al. 2004; Coleman, Parry, Chalmers, & Min, 2006).

Project RED, developed by Jack and colleagues (2009), focuses on a standardized admission and discharge process to assist patients leaving the hospital. A RN discharge advocate provides patient education, medication reconciliation, and coordination for follow-up with the patient's providers. A pharmacist contacts the patient by phone two to four days after discharge and as necessary thereafter. Results found intervention patients experienced lower re-admissions and lower costs at 30 days post-discharge (Strunin, Stone, & Jack, 2007; Jack et al., 2009). EDPP is a telephone-delivered social work interdisciplinary, hospital-to-home intervention developed by Rush University Medical Center, Chicago. Master's prepared social workers (MSW) contact patients approximately two days after discharge. The MSW addresses post-discharge psychosocial and medical issues and follow patients for up to 30 days. Intervention patients had lower 30 day post-discharge mortality rates, higher follow-up physician visits, but no differences in re-admission rates (Perry, Golden, Rooney, & Shier, 2011; Fabbre, Buffington, Altfeld, Shier, & Golden, 2011; Rooney, Markovitz, & Packard, 2011; Altfeld et al., 2013).

Comprehensive Care Coordination

Effective care coordination models include Care Management Plus (CMP), Geriatric Resources and Care for Elders (GRACE), Guided Care, Improving Mood-Promoting Access to Collaborative Treatment (IMPACT), Massachusetts General Hospital Care Management Program (MGH CMP), and the best practice sites from the Medicare Coordinated Care Demonstration (MCCD). Although each model has slightly different components and a different emphasis, they share commonalities in that they:

- Identify patients at high risk of hospitalization in the coming year and improve his/her knowledge of and adherence to treatment and self-care regimes;

- Improve communications and coordination between the patient's PCP and specialists, and these providers and the patient;

- Work with the providers to identify and rectify areas in which care for the patient may not be consistent with evidence-based guidelines;

- Monitor the patient's symptom's, well-being, and adherence between clinical visits;

- Advise the patient on when to see their provider; and

- Notify the patient's PCP of health status change.

CMP, developed by Dorr and colleagues, found that a multi-disease care management program, with RNs located in primary care practices and supported by specialized information technology, was successful in reducing hospitalizations, mortality, and costs for complex diabetic patients (Dorr, Wilcox, Brunker, Burdon, & Donnelly, 2008). There is also evidence that this approach, using specialized clinical information systems to coordinate care for MCC patients, can lead to improved quality of care through rates of adherence to testing guidelines (Dorr, Jones, & Wilcox, 2007). An evaluation of GRACE, a system developed by Counsell and colleagues that provides interdisciplinary team care and home-based care management by a nurse practitioner and social worker, found that it improved quality of care, reduced both overall admissions and readmissions, and resulted in cost savings for a predefined group of low-income at-risk elderly patients (Counsell et al., 2007; Counsell, Callahan, Tu, Stump, & Arling, 2009). Guided Care, developed by Boult and colleagues (2013) and utilizing RNs to enhance primary care practice, demonstrated lower healthcare expenditures, hospitalizations, and emergency department (ED) visits during the initial eight months of the study, but only home healthcare services and cost were significantly reduced at the end of 32 months (Leff et al., 2009; Boult et al. 2013). IMPACT, developed by Unutzer and colleagues, employs a multidisciplinary team approach to depression management, and has demonstrated positive results with depression symptoms for older adults in primary care settings and lower healthcare costs for adults with diabetes (Unutzer et al., 2002; Kanton et al., 2006). Results from MGH CMP, a program developed by Ferris and colleagues that places RN care managers in primary care practices supported by a clinical information system, have shown lower hospitalization and ED rates and lower costs for high risk Medicare beneficiaries (Ferris et al., 2010).

The MCCD, a disease management and care coordination approach to chronic illness care administered by the Centers for Medicare and Medicaid Services (CMS), produced few improvements in quality of care, and only 2 of the 15 original MCCD sites reduced hospitalization rates during 48 months of operation (Peikes, Chen, Schore, & Brown, 2009). However, a secondary analysis of 11 of the original sites over 6 years of operation identified 4 programs (best practice sites) that significantly reduced hospitalization rates by 8 to 33% for a subset of high risk beneficiaries (Gerolamo, Schore, Brown, & Schraeder, 2011; Brown, Peikes, Peterson, Schore, & Razafindrakoto, 2012). When care management fees were included in total costs of care, the programs were essentially cost neutral. One of the best practice sites, Washington University in St. Louis, reduced hospitalizations and monthly Medicare spending in beneficiaries who were much sicker than average Medicare beneficiaries, and almost a third of the enrollees had dual coverage from both Medicare and Medicaid (Peikes, Peterson, Brown, Graff, & Lynch, 2012a). Another best practice site, Health Quality Partners, Doylestown, Pennsylvania, also reduced the risk of all-cause mortality by 25% in the intervention group compared to the control group (Coburn, Marcantonio, Razansky, Keller, & Davis, 2012).

For a concise, in-depth comparison of transitional care models, including program details and outcomes, see Peikes and colleagues (2013) and the National Coalition on Care Coordination (2013). For a detailed review of CMS disease management and care management demonstrations, see Brown and colleagues (2011). See Volland and Wright (2011) and Bozack, Volland, and Weiss (2013) for an overview of integrated social support and long-term care programs.

EFFECTIVE CARE COORDINATION COMPONENTS AND PRACTICES

Based on the results highlighted above, especially the in-depth analyses of the MCCD best practice sites, five components distinguish an effective care coordination intervention (see Table 1).

- *Targeting*: Enrolling patients who will benefit most from the intervention is crucial to program success. MCC individuals with a high likelihood of hospitalization in the year following enrollment are primary candidates to benefit most from the intervention, as opposed to individuals with a high risk for multiple hospitalizations.

- *Staffing*: Longitudinal care should be provided by multidisciplinary teams, with designated RN care managers to deliver the majority of the intervention while being supported by other team members, including social

Table 1 Components of Successful Care Coordination Models

Component	Description
Targeting	Identify patients with select chronic conditions who were hospitalized one or more times in the previous year or at the time of enrollment.
Staffing	Multidisciplinary teams, consisting of the PCP, RN, patient, and other healthcare professionals when necessary (social worker, therapist, pharmacist).
	RN care manager:
	■ Caseload of 40–80 patients
	■ Frequent face-to-face contact with patients (once a month) at home or in clinical setting.
	■ Regular telephone monitoring.
Primary Care Provider Collaboration	Strong rapport with primary care provider/specialist physicians/hospital.
	Regular face-to-face contact through co-location, regular hospital rounds, and accompanying patients on physician visits.
	Assign all of a provider's patients to the same RN care manager.
Information Technology	Patient tracking system.
	Electronic health record components.
	Alert system that notifies RN care manager when patient contacts acute care (ED or hospital).
Training and Feedback	Initial comprehensive training of all team members in care coordination.
	Provide ongoing feedback to care coordination teams on selected processes of care and program outcomes.

workers, rehabilitative therapists, pharmacists, and navigators. Patients should be contacted at least monthly on a face-to-face basis as well as regular telephone monitoring.

■ *Primary care provider collaboration*: Care managers should have regular contact with PCPs, and a PCP's targeted "high risk" patients should be assigned to the same care manager.

■ *Information technology*: A system for documenting care and providing timely information on acute care admissions and ED visits are critical to program effectiveness. This system also interfaces with other systems utilized by the team.

■ *Training and feedback*: All team members should receive initial training in care coordination, and individual care teams should receive regular, specific feedback on overall program outcomes and specific outcomes for their panel of patients.

In addition, effective care coordination interventions share the following activities and practices (see Table 2):

- Follow evidence-based guidelines to manage care;
- Complete a multi-dimensional initial in-home assessment;
- Collaboratively develop and implement a plan of care containing specific action plans and goals with the patient/family and PCP;
- Implement self-care coaching and support, including an effective medication management plan, following evidence-based protocols and models;
- Actively facilitate communication among the patient's providers concerning the patient and his/her health status;
- Monitor and evaluate a patient's symptoms, well-being, and adherence to the plan of care between PCP office visits;
- Manage care setting transitions, especially from hospitals and skilled nursing facilities; and
- Arrange and coordinate needed health-related and community-based support services.

See Schraeder et al. (2011) for a thorough review of effective intervention components, Dorr and King (2011) for an overview of how health information technology can assist in the effective management of MCC, and Newcomer and Dobell (2011) on approaches to evaluate care coordination programs. For a review of successful randomized controlled self-management trials that have demonstrated favorable results with hospitalizations and costs, refer to Lorig and colleagues (1999, 2001), Wheeler (2003), Hibbard and colleagues (2004), and Chodosh et al. (2005).

THE NURSING ROLE IN EFFECTIVE CARE COORDINATION

The successful care coordination models discussed above utilized RNs as the primary providers of the intervention, reinforcing evidence that enhanced and integral involvement of RNs in the coordination and delivery of care for patients with MCC is critical to positive cost and quality outcomes (Fisher et al., 2009), and that nursing is paramount to the delivery of high-quality care (Naylor et al., 2013). A recent IOM report (2011) suggests that nurses will need to practice to the full extent of their education and training to coordinate increasingly complex care for a wide range of patients, fulfilling their potential as primary care providers by working in collaborative teams focused on the patient's unique set of needs.

Table 2 Successful Care Coordination Practices and Activities

Practice/Activity	Description
Evidence-based guidelines (national or developed internally by committee and updated annually)	■ Guidelines that cover medical care, nursing care, patient/family education, and self-management. ■ Chronic conditions: CHF, diabetes, COPD, CAD. ■ Self-care activities: glucose checks, daily weights, blood pressure logs, exercise, proper nutrition, etc. ■ Syndromes: falls, hydration, incontinence, sleep, substance use. ■ Health promotion activities: immunizations, mammograms, colonoscopy, etc.
Comprehensive assessment	■ Initial face-to-face meeting in the home, office, or hospital. ■ Domains: demographics, medical history, cognition, psychosocial (nutrition, sleep, substance use), functional status (medication management, self-care), environmental, safety, caregiver assessment.
Care plan development	■ Patient centered and patient directed (mutual goals and action plans). ■ Identification of red flags that signal worsening condition. ■ Proactive monitoring at predetermined intervals or in anticipation of change in health status. ■ Patient education/education to increase self-management skills. ■ Medication management (reconciliation with care transitions, pharmacist review, affordability issues, between multiple provider visits). ■ Identify and address gaps and barriers to care.
Care plan implementation, monitoring, and evaluation	■ Frequency of contacts determined at predetermined intervals for further assessment, teaching/coaching and monitoring of self-management activities, and evaluating effectiveness of care plan. ■ Monitoring schedule based on patient's chronic illnesses, recommendations from guidelines, PCP feedback, self-management activities, current medications, service utilization history, and patient/caregiver preference. ■ Patient/caregiver contact care manager with any change in health status. ■ Referrals can be made to address patient/caregiver needs and evaluate effectiveness of services
Self-management	■ Assess patient/caregivers: current level of self-care ability, health literacy, readiness to change, problem-solving abilities. ■ Teach/coach on needed strategies and activities: information on community-based education/support groups, written material based on guidelines, life-style modification to improve control of conditions, health promotion/maintenance needs. ■ End-of-life teaching to include advance directives.
Medication management	■ Assess medications at each contact (recent changes, perceived effectiveness, adverse reactions, adherence, difficulty obtaining or affording). ■ Consult with pharmacist and/or PCP to discuss possible problems and address barriers to adherence. ■ Provide education on the purpose of the medication(s), expected therapeutic effects, side effects to monitor for, and report to appropriate provider.

(continued)

Practice/Activity	Description
Transitional care	■ Occurs any time the patient moves across the continuum of care: home to hospital, hospital to nursing facility, back to hospital or discharge home.
	■ Frequently accompanied by changes in status, medication, or self-management needs.
	■ Care managers follow patients across the continuum of care and continue to provide education, medication reconciliation, communication between providers, coaching on self-management needs, home and community assessments, and coordination of referrals as needed.
	■ Care managers contact discharge planners and other service providers to identify discharge and service needs.
	■ Patients are visited soon after admission or within first few days after discharge.
Information technology	■ Supports care coordination by bridging gaps and enhancing communication:
	● Secure electronic messaging system
	● Alerts about test results
	● Notification of reviews from other team members
	● Access to medical records
	● Notification of inpatient or ED admission
	● Generate reminders for contacts, testing, health promotion needs, follow-up with PCP or specialty providers
	● Ensure updated medication lists are available to all team members
	● Patient-focused websites that provide patient information and education
Program evaluation	■ Intervention structure and implementation:
	● Adherence to and implementation of guidelines and protocols
	● Decreased medication management issues
	● Improved self-management skills
	● Increased use of health prevention services
	■ Quality related processes:
	● Improved patient quality of life
	● Patient and provider satisfaction
	■ Healthcare utilization and cost measures:
	● Prevention of avoidable hospitalizations and re-hospitalizations
	● Decreased hospital days

The care coordination role is vastly different from that of primary care nursing or home health nursing. Care coordination is a complex task and the RN care manager has multiple roles to play, such as:

■ Developing and maintaining collaborative relationships within a multidisciplinary primary care team;

- Developing an individualized care plan with the patient and their caregiver in collaboration with other team members based upon their goals, strengths, and current needs;

- Working with patients and their caregiver in goal setting and prioritizing care that is both appropriate and safe;

- Educating and coaching patients and their caregiver using adult learning concepts and principles about their health conditions, medications, "red flags," and self-management tasks;

- Coordinating and evaluating care provided by other health and community providers;

- Evaluating care provided and adjusting the plan of care as needed;

- Updating team members and other health and community providers about changes in the patient's health status; and

- During transitions in care, facilitating communication between health and community providers, and between the patient and caregiver and their providers.

Effective care coordination shifts the responsibility of care management decision-making to a collaborative relationship between the patient and the primary care team. Within this paradigm shift, care managers must learn their new roles within the work environment culture, which includes team member skills and personalities, and the day-to-day flow of the clinical setting so that the model can enhance, rather than duplicate or threaten, current operations. The challenge for the care manager is to create a role that works to fill in the gaps and improve chronic illness through collaborative practice.

SKILLS NEEDED FOR EFFECTIVE CARE COORDINATION

Effective care coordination starts with nurses, physicians, and ancillary healthcare providers learning and practicing care coordination. Care coordination requires specific skills, especially in the areas of collaboration, interpersonal communication, and teamwork. Skills in these areas allow providers to integrate actions and expertise, negotiate judgment differences through timely transfer of accurate clinical information, and determine shared roles and priorities for patient care as opposed to individual clinical providers (Press, Michelow, & MacPhail, 2012). Many healthcare professionals lack the education and preparation necessary to coordinate care for patients in rapidly changing healthcare settings and an evolving healthcare system (Pham, O'Malley, Bach, Salontz-Martinez, & Schrag, 2009).

There is a shortage of RNs with sufficient training and experience in the clinical practice and team management skills that effective care coordination requires. It has been suggested that more nurses need further education and training in the management of complex health conditions and coordination of care with multiple health professionals. RNs need to acquire new competencies in systems thinking, quality improvement, care management, and a basic understanding of health policy and research principles (Sochalski & Weiner, 2010).

What are the essential skills nurses need to participate in the development of effective care programs; to deliver high quality care that is patient-centered, evidence-based, sustainable, and cost effective at the appropriate time? Below is a brief list and description of these skills.

- Population health management (PHM): Effective care coordination calls for a change from a focus on a single provider caring for the health and well-being of an individual patient to a focus on a healthcare team managing the health of a panel of patients. The goal of PHM is to keep a patient population as healthy as possible, minimizing the need for extensive interventions and procedures. PHM encompasses defining a patient population, identifying gaps in care, stratifying risks, engaging patients in the management of their care, and measuring outcomes at the patient population level (Felt-Lisk & Higgins, 2011).

- Comprehensive Assessment and Care Planning: A thorough knowledge of chronic disease management and evidence-based guidelines and protocols, especially for CHF, COPD, diabetes, and depression. A dual diagnosis of diabetes and depression is common in the elderly and often leads to poor health and utilization outcomes (McSharry, Bishop, Moss-Morris, & Kendrick, 2013).

- Interpersonal communication: Includes the ability to use different communication styles, including active listening, to counsel, interview, resolve conflict, build relationships, and develop effective interdisciplinary teams. An understanding of family and group dynamics is essential for developing collaborative relationships and team care.

- Education/coaching: A working knowledge of adult education principles and learning techniques, readiness to change, and identification of necessary person-centered components for a self-management plan is necessary to overcome barriers to patient and caregiver learning and facilitate behavior change.

- Health insurance and benefits: Must have current knowledge of health insurance, managed care, and other payer sources and benefits. This includes specific information on public (e.g., Medicare, Medicaid, SSI, SSDI, VA) and private (e.g., pharmacy benefit programs, employer sponsored health coverage, individual insurance policies, home care benefits) program benefits.

- Community resources: A thorough familiarity of public and private community-based providers, services, and support available in the local geographical area.

- Research and evaluation: A basic understanding of research and evaluation techniques to assist in quality improvement of care and interpretation of program outcomes and effectiveness. Specific areas include: collecting, analyzing, and synthesizing population outcome data; evaluating the quality of patient education materials; identifying research-substantiated, evidence-based guidelines and interventions for the ongoing care needs of chronically ill patients; having an understanding of appropriate statistical methods for analyzing interventional components and program outcomes; staying current with the care management, case management, and disease management literature; and writing skills for proposals that fund additional research program reports. Skills for writing manuscripts/articles for publication in nursing and other health related journals to disseminate program results are essential for program growth and professional development.

MOVING TOWARD EFFECTIVE CARE COORDINATION

The U.S. healthcare system is slowly changing the way care is delivered. Changes are being propelled at the federal level, as well as through public and private partnerships to start preparing for payment changes from fee-for-service reimbursement. At the federal level, three legislative provisions in the Affordable Care Act, the Hospital Readmissions Reduction Program, the National Pilot Program on Payment Bundling, and the Community-Based Care Transitions Program, administered by the Center for Medicare and Medicaid Innovation (CMMI), are designed to enhance care transitions for Medicare beneficiaries coping with chronic illnesses. Public and private organizations are supporting PCMHs and ACOs as well. The reimbursement system that will replace fee-for-service is still in the making, but it will certainly include increased financial and clinical accountability.

Although the programs mentioned above do not have a long shelf life, valuable lessons are already being learned. Despite the potential of the three federal programs to reduce fragmentation and increase care coordination, red flags are already being raised because effective program implementation and replication may take a back seat to reducing hospitalizations and costs (Naylor et al., 2012). PCMHs and ACOs are evolving rapidly, and early results are promising in reducing unnecessary hospital and ED utilization, but the results are mostly inconclusive (Peikes et al., 2012b). However, results indicate several trends and insight into the evolving nature of care coordination: (1) a strong foundation is needed for successful transformation, especially information technology capability; (2) transformation is a long and difficult journey and does not happen overnight, it requires time and effort; and (3) although approaches to transformation vary, an emphasis on team-based care is essential for expanded access and improved coordination, and data-driven measurement and feedback are the foundation of quality improvement (McNellis, Genevro, & Meyers, 2013; Sinsky et al., 2013).

Responding to the deficiencies in chronic care management for Medicare beneficiaries, the CMS has implemented the triple aim of improving individual health, improving population health, and decreasing healthcare costs. Unfortunately, despite the logic for and evidence base behind the care coordination models discussed above, results have not provided convincing evidence that any one model can achieve all three goals. As effective care coordination models are developed and implemented, there will be a pressing need to further understand the "black box" of the intervention. Research should be conducted which increases understanding of the following: which high-risk population to target at different age levels in order to produce cost-effective outcomes; the optimal duration of the intervention; the type and duration of contacts with patients and team members; the care coordination emphasis (i.e., assessing, planning, coaching, monitoring, and evaluating); the mix of components (medical care and social service supports) of collaborative person-centered care and joint decision-making; development and use of evidence-based self-management protocols combined with effective delivery methods; identification and utilization of effective information technology tools with patients, their caregivers, and team members; and how to evaluate and educate the care coordination team and its individual members in implementing a cost-effective care coordination intervention.

The evidence indicates that the CMMI should administer and evaluate a coordinated care intervention that has the best chance of achieving the goal of improving quality of care for Medicare beneficiaries with chronic illnesses while reducing utilization of expensive healthcare services. The proposed coordinated care demonstration would build on the evidence from prior CMS demonstrations and successful care coordination programs to identify whom to serve and what to deliver. Taking the lessons learned, restricting the eligible population to those proven to benefit, developing protocols to tightly specify the intervention, basing decisions on actual experience, and testing the replicability of favorable past results in other settings is a logical next step to build on CMS's earlier investments in changing care delivery. The demonstration would test this replicability within a short time period to give CMS concrete lessons about how a successful care coordination model might be disseminated more broadly.

The proposed demonstration would involve 10 to 12 sites in geographically different regions of the country. All participating sites would implement the same standardized intervention and target the same high-risk subgroup of Medicare beneficiaries with chronic conditions who are likely to undergo expensive care in the absence of an intervention. The demonstration would replicate care coordination strategies that have been found to be successful in the evaluation of the MCCD. The intervention would utilize care coordination protocols developed jointly, or national guidelines adopted by all participating sites. RN care managers would interact on a routine basis with patients, their PCPs, and other health/social service providers as part of the intervention protocol. The RN care managers would have the primary responsibility for executing processes according to protocol. The demonstration would cover a period of four years, including 6 to 12 months for enrollment of a minimum number of participants required for the study and random assignment into treatment or control groups, and a full four-year operational period from program startup to study end.

This demonstration would be evaluated from three different perspectives. The first would be an impact analysis, which would document the operations of each national site. A specific focus of the implementation study would be documenting how and why each site adapted the evidence-based protocols to its unique context, and how faithful actual implementation was to the planned program model. The second perspective would consist of an impact analysis, using Medicare enrollment, claims data, and patient survey data to estimate program effects on Medicare expenditures and service use, mortality, patient adherence to recommended self-care regimes, patient satisfaction, and quality-of-life indicators and measures. The third perspective would consist of drawing inferences from the implementation findings and impact estimates to draw inferences about program structure and processes that contributed to any improved patient, quality, or cost outcomes, as well as lessons learned for broad dissemination of the program model. Refer to Table 3 for specifics of the proposed demonstration.

Table 3 Proposed Care Coordination Demonstration Parameters

Demonstration Parameters	Description
Sample research questions	■ How is the intervention implemented in different settings? ■ Does it change patients' self-care behaviors? ■ Does it improve patients' well-being (quality of life)? ■ What do patients and PCPs think of the intervention? ■ Does it generate net savings to Medicare and improve care quality? ■ What program and organizational features are most strongly associated with positive impacts? ■ What fee levels would cover the intervention costs and still yield net savings to Medicare?
National sites	■ Commitment: Four year intervention, five year evaluation ■ 12 national sites (different geographical regions) ■ Possible selection criteria: 　● Capacity to implement (infrastructure, personnel, data systems) 　● Ability to identify and enroll eligible beneficiaries 　● History of working collaboratively with other sites or research teams 　● Length of the demonstration and number of sites to be negotiated with CMS.
Patient eligibility criteria	■ Medicare as primary payer (enrolled in Parts A and B). ■ Live within a defined service area. ■ Not enrolled in hospice care or Part C, not residing in LTC facility for more than 90 days, not ESRD. ■ High Risk Criteria: 　● Diagnosed with CHF, CAD, and/or COPD and a hospitalization in past year.
Site enrollment	■ Enroll at least 800 beneficiaries within first 6 to 12 months of program setup. ■ Voluntary enrollment and disenrollment. ■ Random assignment to intervention or control group by household. ■ 60:40 treatment-control enrollment ratio enables sites to reach sustainable size quicker (also less discouraging for referral sources).
Core intervention components	■ Clinical assessment: standardized, comprehensive, initial in-home. ■ Evidence-based guidelines and protocols: CHF, CAD, COPD, geriatric problems (falls, incontinence, depression). ■ Care planning: mutual, prioritized goals/action plans. ■ Care plan implementation: self-management strategies, service/provider coordination, reporting changes in symptoms, medications, self-management activities. ■ Patient and family monitoring. ■ Care plan evaluation.

Demonstration Parameters	Description

Core intervention components (continued)	■ Special emphasis on:
	  ● Transitional care
	  ● Self-management skills and behaviors
	  ● Medication management
	  ● Collaboration with physicians and other health/community providers.

Intervention staffing	■ RNs as care coordinators with patients and their families/caregiver. ■ Coordination with PCP and other health/community providers. ■ Patient panel: 80 to 100.
Core information system components	■ Individual care plan/protocols. ■ Clinical patient summary. ■ Basic prioritization of patient. ■ Care coordinator activities. ■ Patient/provider reminders. ■ Interactive goal-setting form/template. ■ Structured encounter form. ■ Quality reports. ■ Comprehensive list of patient's medications. ■ Patient database: patient risk stratification. ■ Eligibility determination process. ■ Record of care coordinator contacts with PCP. ■ Electronic social support resources.

Evaluation approaches	■ Process Evaluation:
	  ● Descriptive site analysis
	  ● Implementation assessment
	  ● Fidelity assessment.
	■ Impact Analysis:
	  ● General and disease specific
	  ● Process of care
	  ● Clinical care
	  ● Care outcomes: health behaviors, health and functional status, patient satisfaction
	  ● Total Medicare costs for Part A and B services, with and without program fees
	  ● Use by type of service: hospitalizations, home health, hospice, outpatient services, ED, physician services, SNF admissions.
	■ Synthesis Evaluation:
	  ● Variations in impacts across sites
	  ● Exploratory analysis across individual sites
	  ● Lessons learned.

(continued)

Demonstration Parameters	Description
Sample key policy questions	■ Would a permanent care coordination option for selected beneficiaries benefit both Medicare and participants?
	■ What care coordination model features are most important?
	■ What operational protocols for programs and their care coordinators should be required?
	■ What types of organizations are best suited to provide effective care coordination in Medicare fee-for-service?
	■ Would changes in eligibility increase savings?
	■ What monthly fees would yield savings to Medicare and cover costs of effective care coordination?

SUMMARY

As the U.S. healthcare system moves slowly toward delivery and payment transformation, the needs of individuals with multiple chronic conditions, who account for the majority of annual healthcare spending, highlight the pressing need for more effective approaches to care coordination. Transformation involves moving from paying for service volume to ongoing coordination of patient care to realize improved quality and health outcomes. Transformation requires a primary care workforce with different clinical and managerial skills that focus on team-based care delivery and population health management. The evidence indicates that the current healthcare workforce does not have the necessary training and skills to accomplish this daunting task.

This chapter has provided a brief overview of the best-practice evidence on care coordination, program components necessary to provide effective care coordination, and the skills needed to function in team-based care coordination. Despite the evidence, replicating interventions that proved successful in a controlled research environment can be difficult in the real world; conditions vary greatly among different care settings, patient populations, and provider organizations. New evidence is needed to confirm the best practice care coordination strategies presented in this chapter. It is suggested that CMMI consider a demonstration of the magnitude outlined above as the best chance of achieving the triple aim of improving individual health, improving population health, and decreasing healthcare costs for the Medicare program. Nurses are at the center of effective care coordination. It is recommended that nursing take the lead in forming collaborative, interdisciplinary relationships with other healthcare professions to contribute much needed evidence to the national policy debate through the implementation and evaluation of an effective care coordination demonstration for chronically ill Americans.

REFERENCES

Altfeld, S. J., Shier, G. E., Rooney, M., Johnson, T. J., Golden, R. L., Karavolos, … Perry, A. J. (2013). Effects of an enhanced discharged planning intervention on hospitalized older adults: A randomized trial. *The Gerontologist, 53,* 430–440.

Anderson, G. (2010). *Chronic care: Making the case for ongoing care.* Princeton, NJ: Robert Wood Johnson Foundation. Retrieved from http://www.rwjf.org/files/research/50968chronic.care.chartbook.pdf

Berwick, D. M., & Hackbarth, A. D. (2012). Eliminating waste in U.S. health care. *Journal of the American Medical Association, 307,* 1513–1516.

Bettger, J. P., Alexander, K. P., Dolor, R. J., Olson, D. M., Kendrick, A. S., Wing, … Duncan, P. W. (2012). Transitional care after hospitalization for acute stroke or myocardial infarction: A systematic review. *Annals of Internal Medicine, 157,* 407–416.

Blumenthal, D. (2012). Performance improvement in health care – seizing the moment. *The New England Journal of Medicine, 366,* 1953–1955.

Boult, C., Leff, B., Boyd, C. M., Wolff, J. L., Marsteller, J. A., Frick, K. D., Wegner, S. et al. (2013). A matched-pair cluster-randomized trial of guided care for high-risk older patients. *Journal of General Internal Medicine.* doi: 10.1007/s11606-012-2287-y

Bozack, A., Volland, P., & Weiss, L. (2013). Expanding research on care coordination for older adults: A discussion of programs, methods, and outcomes. *Policy, Research, & Practice, Issue Brief, 1*(1), New York Academy of Medicine. Retrieved from http://www.nyam.org/news/publications/research-and-reports/Online-Issue-Brief/HTML/issue-brief.htm

Brown, R. (2009). *The promise of care coordination: Models that decrease hospitalizations and improve outcomes for Medicare beneficiaries with chronic illnesses.* New York, NY: New York Academy of Medicine, Social Work Leadership Institute, National Coalition on Care Coordination.

Brown, R. S., Ghosh, A., Schraeder, C., & Shelton, P. (2011). Promising practices in acute/primary care. In C. Schraeder & P. Shelton (Eds.), *Comprehensive care coordination for chronically ill adults* (pp. 39–64). West Sussex, UK: John Wiley & Sons.

Brown, R. S., Peikes, D., Peterson, G., Schore, J., & Razafindrakoto, C. M. (2012). Six features of Medicare coordinated care demonstration programs that cut hospital admissions of high risk patients. *Health Affairs, 31,* 1156–1166.

Coburn, K. D., Marcantonio, S., Lazansky, R., Keller, M., & Davis, N. (2012). Effect of a community-based nursing intervention on mortality in chronically ill older adults: A randomized controlled trial. *PLoS Medicine, 9*(7), e1001265. doi: 10.1371/journal.pmed.1001265

Codosh, J., Morton, S. C., Mojica, W., Maglione, M., Suttorp, M. J., Hilton, … Shekelle, P. (2005). Meta-analysis: Chronic disease self-management programs for older adults. *Annals of Internal Medicine, 143:*427–438.

Coleman, E. A., Smith, J. D., Frank, J. C., Min, S., Parry, C., & Kramer, A. M. (2004). Preparing patients and caregivers to participate in care delivered across settings: The care transitions intervention. *Journal of the American Geriatrics Society, 52,* 1817–1825.

Coleman, E. A., Parry, C., Chalmers, S., & Min, S. J. (2006). The care transitions intervention: Results of a randomized controlled trial. *Archives of Internal Medicine, 166,* 1822–1828.

Coleman, K., Austin, B. T., Brach, C., & Wagner, E. H. (2009). Evidence on the chronic care model in the new millennium. *Health Affairs, 28*(1), 75–85.

Counsell, S. R., Callahan, C. M., Clark, D. O., Tu, W., Buttar, A. B., Stump, T. E., & Ricketts, G. D. (2007). Geriatric care management for low-income seniors: A randomized controlled trial. *Journal of the American Medical Association, 298,* 2623–2633.

Counsell, S. R., Callahan, C. M., Tu, W., Stump, T. E., & Arling, G. W. (2009). Cost analysis of the geriatric resources for assessment and care of elders care management intervention. *Journal of the American Geriatrics Society, 57,* 1420–1426.

de Bruin, S. R., Versnel, N., Lemmens, L. C., Molema, C. C. M., Schellevis, F. G., Nijpels, G., & Baan, C. A. (2012). Comprehensive care programs for patients with multiple chronic conditions: A systematic literature review. *Health Policy, 107*(2–3), 108–145.

Dorr, D. A., Jones, S. S., & Wilcox, A. (2007). A framework for information system usage in collaborative care. *Journal of Biomedical Informatics, 40,* 282–287.

Dorr, D. A., Wilxom, A. B., Brunker, C. P., Burdon, R. E., & Donnelly, S. M. (2008). The effect of technology-supported, multidisease care management on the mortality and hospitalization of seniors. *Journal of the American Geriatrics Society, 56,* 2195–2202.

Dorr, D. A., & King, M. M. (2011). Health information technology. In C. Schraeder & P. Shelton (Eds.), *Comprehensive care coordination for chronically ill adults* (pp. 141–165). West Sussex, UK: John Wiley & Sons.

Fabbre, V. D., Buffington, A. S., Altfeld, S. J., Shier, G. E., & Golden, R. L. (2011). Social work and transitions of care: Observations from an intervention for older adults. *Journal of Gerontological Social Work, 54,* 615–626.

Felt-Liks, S., & Higgins, T. (2011). Issue brief: Exploring the promise of population health management programs to improve health. Washington, DC: Mathematica Policy Research, Inc. Retrieved from http://www.mathematica-mpr.com/publications/pdfs/health/PHM_brief.pdf

Ferris, T. G., Weil, E., Meyer, G. S., Neagle, M., Heffernan, J. L., & Torchiana, D. F. (2010). Cost savings from managing high-risk patients. In National Research Council, *The healthcare imperative: Lowering costs and improving outcomes. Workshop series summary* (pp. 301–310). Washington, DC: National Academies Press.

Fisher, E. S., McClellan, M. B., Bertko, J., Lieberman, S. M., Lee, J. J., Lewis, L., & Skinner, J. S. (2009). Fostering accountable health care: Moving forward in Medicare. *Health Affairs, 28,* w219–w231.

Gerolamo, A. M., Schore, J., Brown, R. S., & Schraeder, C. (2011). Medicare coordinated care. In In C. Schraeder & P. Shelton (Eds.), *Comprehensive care coordination for chronically ill adults* (pp. 229–259). West Sussex, UK: John Wiley & Sons.

Hassen, L. O., Young, R. S., Hinami, K., Leung, A., & Williams, M. V. (2011). Interventions to reduce 30-day rehospitalization: A systematic review. *Annals of Internal Medicine, 155,* 520–528.

Hibbard, J. H., Stockard, J., Mahoney, E. R., & Tusler, M. (2004). Development of the patient activation measure (PAM): Conceptualizing and measuring activation in patients and consumers. *Health Services Research, 39*(4, Part I), 1005–1026.

Institute of Medicine (IOM). (2001). *Crossing the quality chasim: A new health system for the twenty-first century.* Washington, DC: National Academies Press.

Institute of Medicine (IOM). (2010). *The future of nursing: Leading change, advancing health.* Washington, DC: National Academies Press.

Jack, B. W., Chetty, V. P., Anthony, D., Greenwald, J. L., Sanchez, G. M., Johnson, A. E., Forsythe, S. R., et al. (2009). A reengineered hospital discharge program to decrease rehospitalization: A randomized trial. *Annals of Internal Medicine, 150,* 178–187.

Kanton, W. J., Unutzer, J., Fan, M. Y., Williams, J., Schoenbaum, M., Lin, E., & Hunkeler, E. (2006). Cost-effectiveness and net benefit of enhanced treatment of depression for older adults with diabetes and depression. *Diabetes Care, 29,* 265–270.

Keehan, S. P., Sisko, A. M., Truffer, C. J., Poisal, J. A., Cuckler, G. A., Madison, A. J., ... Smith, S. D. (2011). National health spending projections through 2020: Economic recovery and reform drive faster spending growth. *Health Affairs, 30,* 1594–1605.

Leff, B., Reider, L., Frick, K. D., Scharfstein, D. O., Boyd, C. M., Frey, K., ... Boult, C. (2009). Guided care and the cost of complex healthcare: A preliminary report. *American Journal of Managed Care, 15,* 555–559.

Lorig, K. R., Sobel, D. S., Stewart, A. L., Brown, B. W., Bandura, A., Ritter, P., ... Holman, H. R. (1999). Evidence suggesting that a chronic disease self-management program can improve health status while reducing hospitalization: A randomized trial. *Medical Care, 37*(1), 5–14.

Lorig, K. R., Ritter, P., Stewart, A. L., Sobel, D. S., Brown, B. W., Bandura, A., ... Holman, H. R. (2001). Chronic disease self-management program: 2-year health status and health care utilization outcomes. *Medical Care, 39,* 1217–1223.

McNellis, R. J., Genevro, J. L., & Meyers, D. S. (2013). Lessons learned from the study of primary care transformation. *Annals of Family Medicine, 11*(Suppl 1), S1–S5.

McSharry, J., Bishop, F. L., Moss-Morris, R., & Kendrick, T. (2013). 'The chicken and egg thing': Cognitive representations and self-management of multimorbidity in people with diabetes and depression. *Psychology & Health, 28*(1), 103–119.

Naylor, M. D., Brooten, D., Campbell, R., Jacobsen, B. S., Mezey, M. D., Pauly, M. V., & Schwartz, J. S. (1999). Comprehensive discharge planning and home follow-up of hospitalized elders: A randomized clinical trial. *Journal of the American Medical Association, 281,* 613–620.

Naylor, M. D., Brooten, D. A., Campbell, R. L., Maislin, G., McCauley, K. M., & Schwartz, J. S. (2004). Transitional care of older adults hospitalized with heart failure: A randomized, controlled trial. *Journal of the American Geriatrics Society, 52,* 675–684.

Naylor, M. D., Kurtzman, E. T., Grabowski, D. C., Harrington, C., McClellan, M., & Reinard, S. C. (2012). Unintended consequences of steps to cut readmissions and reform payment may threaten care of vulnerable older adults. *Health Affairs, 31,* 1623–1632.

Naylor, M. D., Volpe, E. M., Lustig, A., Kelley, H. J., Melichar, L., & Pauly, M. V. (2013). Linkages between nursing and the quality of patient care: A 2-year comparison. *Medical Care, 51*(Suppl 2), S6–S14.

National Coalition on Care Coordination (2013). Issue brief: Care coordination. Retrieved from http://www.eldercareworkforce.org/research/issue-briefs/research:care-coordination-brief/

Newcomer, R., & Dobell, L. G. (2011). Evaluation methods. In C. Schraeder & P. Shelton (Eds.), *Comprehensive care coordination for chronically ill adults* (pp. 127–140). West Sussex, UK: John Wiley & Sons.

Parekh, A. K., & Barton, M. B. (2010). The challenge of multiple comorbodity for the U.S. health care system. *Journal of the American Medical Association, 303,* 1303–1304.

Peikes, D., Chen, A., Schore, J., & Brown, R. (2009). Effects of care coordination on hospitalization, quality of care, and health care expenditures among Medicare beneficiaries: 15 randomized trials. *Journal of the American Medical Association, 301,* 603–618.

Peikes, D., Peterson, G., Brown, R. S., Graff, S., & Lynch, J. P. (2012a). How changes in Washington University's Medicare coordinated care demonstration pilot ultimately achieved savings. *Health Affairs, 31,* 1216–1226.

Peikes, D., Zutshi, A., Genevro, J., Smith, K., Parchman, M., & Meyers, D. (2012b). *Early evidence on the patient-centered medical home. Final Report.* Rockville, MD: Agency for Healthcare Research and Quality, Publication No. 12-0020-EF.

Peikes, D., Lester, R. S., Gilman, B., & Brown, R. (2013). The effects of transitional care models on re-admissions: A review of the current evidence. *Generations, 36*(4), 44–55.

Perry, A. J., Golden, R. L., Rooney, M., & Shier, G. E. (2011). Enhanced discharge planning program at Rush University medical center. In C. Schraeder & P. Shelton (Eds.), *Comprehensive care coordination for chronically ill adults* (pp. 277–290). West Sussex, UK: John Wiley & Sons.

Pham, H. H., O'Malley, A. S., Bach, P. B., Salontz-Martinez, C., & Schrag, D. (2009). Primary care physicians' links to other physicians through Medicare patients: The scope of care coordination. *Annals of Internal Medicine, 150,* 236–242.

Press, M. J., Michelow, M. D., & MacPhail, L. H. (2012). Care coordination in accountable care organizations: Moving beyond structure and incentives. *American Journal of Managed Care, 18,* 778–780.

Reuben, D. B. (2007). Better care for older people with chronic diseases: An emerging vision. *Journal of the American Medical Association, 298,* 2673–2674.

Rooney, M., Markovitz, D., & Packard, M. (2011). The enhanced discharge planning program eases a patient's transition home. *Generations, 35*(4), 78–80.

Schimpff, S. C. (2012). *The future of health-care delivery: Why it must change and how it will affect you*. Washington, DC: Potomac Books.

Schraeder, C., Brunker, C. P., Hess, I., Hale, B. A., Berger, C., & Waldschmidt, V. (2011). Intervention components. In C. Schraeder & P. Shelton (Eds.), *Comprehensive care coordination for chronically ill adults* (pp. 87–126). West Sussex, UK: John Wiley & Sons.

Sinsky, C. A., Willard-Grace, R., Schutzbank, A. M., Sinsky, T. A., Margolius, D., & Bodenheimer, T. (2013). In search of joy in practice: A report of 23 high-functioning primary care practices. *Annals of Family Medicine*, 11, 272–278.

Sochalski, J., & Weiner, J. (2010). Health care system reform and the nursing workforce: Matching nursing practice and skills to future needs, not past demands. In Institute of Medicine, *The future of nursing: Leading change, advancing health* (pp. 375–400). Washington, DC: National Academies Press.

Strunin, L., Stone, M., & Jack, B. Understanding rehospitalization risk: Can the hospital discharge be modified to impact recurrent hospitalization? *Journal of Hospital Medicine*, 2, 297–304.

Tinetti, M. E., Fried, T. R., & Boyd, C. M. (2012). Designing health care for the most common chronic condition – multimorbidity. *Journal of the American Medical Association*, 307, 2493–2494.

Unutzer, J., Katon, W., Callahan, C. M., Williams, J. W., Hunkeler, E., Harpole, L., et al. (2002). Collaborative care management of late-life depression in the primary care setting: A randomized controlled trial. *Journal of the American Medical Association*, 288, 2836–2845.

Vogeli, C., Shields, A. E., Lee, T. A., Gibson, T. B., Marder, W. D., Weiss, K. B., & Blumenthal, D. (2007). Multiple chronic conditions: Prevalence, health consequences, and implications for quality, care management, and costs. *Journal of General Internal Medicine*, 22(Suppl. 3), 391–395.

Volland, P. J., & Wright, M. E. (2011). Promising practices in integrated care. In C. Schraeder & P. Shelton (Eds.), *Comprehensive care coordination for chronically ill adults* (pp. 65–86). West Sussex, UK: John Wiley & Sons.

Ward, B. W., & Schiller, J. S. (2013). Prevalence of multiple chronic conditions among U.S. adults: Estimates from the National Health Interview Survey, 2010. *Preventing Chronic Disease*, 10, 120203. http://dx.doi.org/10.5888/pcd10.120203

Wheeler, J. (2003). Can a disease self-management program reduce health care costs? The case of older women with heart disease. *Medical Care*, 41, 706–715.

Chapter 5

Recognizing Care Coordination in Nurses' Practice

Gerri Lamb, PhD, RN, FAAN; Madeline Schmitt, PhD, RN, FAAN; and Daryl Sharp, PhD, PMHCNS-BC, NPP

The emphasis on care coordination roles has increased with the recognition that improved care coordination is essential in achieving the "Triple Aim" (IHI, 2013) of improved patient experience and improved population health at lower costs. In efforts to identify priority areas for improving the quality of care, better care coordination was identified as a one of two national priority "cross-cutting" areas believed to be relevant to 18 specific areas of health care, e.g., asthma, diabetes, hypertension, and major depression (IOM, 2003). More recently, it has become a required characteristic of the certified patient-centered medical home model in primary care (NCQA, 2011) and a centerpiece of the CMS Accountable Care Organization model for Medicare patients (CMS, 2013.).

However, care coordination has been part of nursing practice since the very beginning of the profession (IOM, 2010). Whereas the previous chapters document the growth in interest in care coordination in health care and nursing, as well as the wealth of different models that have emerged over the years, the purpose of this chapter is to identify nurse care coordination activities in daily practice in order to heighten awareness of this important work and illuminate opportunities for nurses to own and improve their care coordination functions.

Nurses in all practice settings carry out essential care coordination activities. Although the impetus and context for care coordination have changed with significant shifts in our healthcare system and its priorities, the emphasis of care coordination has remained centered on addressing patient needs and preferences through timely and effective communication and care planning. These are activities that are embedded in the day-to-day and moment-to-moment work of nurses in collaboration with their team members.

In contrast to nurses and others for whom care coordination is a primary role function, nurses in *all* other roles—the bedside nurse in the hospital; the home healthcare nurse; the nurse in a nursing home, rehabilitation facility, or dialysis center; the nurse practitioner in a primary care clinic—practice care coordination as part of their diverse and complex work. For example, in a study cited in the IOM (2010) report, *The Future of Nursing*, Lamb and colleagues (2011) found that hospital staff nurses engage in six care coordination activities on a daily basis. Many nurses do not recognize they are performing vital care coordination activities for patients and families. (See the sidebar on page 83 for a short exercise about this.)

MAKING CARE COORDINATION VISIBLE IN NURSING PRACTICE

What difference does it make if a nurse identifies care coordination activities especially if he or she is doing them anyway? You might think that the benefits of care coordination will be accomplished even if the nurse, patient, or anyone else on the healthcare team does not make those activities explicit to themselves or others. There are a number of excellent arguments with supporting research to counter this view. First, consider the implications of non-reflective practice. Nurses may be doing some or all care coordination activities; however, in the absence of the systematic scrutiny and evaluation that comes with reflective activity, it is unlikely that these practices are carried out as effectively and efficiently as required within a coordinated plan of care. Care coordination, as we have seen in earlier chapters, is complicated. Like much of the work of nurses, care coordination requires exquisite integration of patient needs and preferences into a collaboratively developed plan. Then, care coordination involves making sure that the plan gets modified as necessary and carried out across multiple stakeholders at the right place and time. Nurses' inability to reflect on and make explicit the care coordination activities that are part of their work may leave critical holes in the care plan, leading to poorer short and longer term outcomes. Research by Ebright (2004) and Gurses, Carayon, and Wall (2009) mapping the cognitive work of nurses indicates that if nurses do not understand their work, the result is adverse quality for patients. Ebright underscores the drawbacks of not fully identifying or understanding what we do.

> *System experts have taught us that failure to understand the work of care providers in actual caregiving situations is a major stumbling point in making real progress. Recently published research on the characteristics of nursing work identifies it as highly complex. Much of the complexity is due to the need for nurses*

to manage highly complicated processes and environmental issues in the midst of delivering individualized care. (Ebright, 2004, p.168)

More specifically, as you will read in the next section of this book, poor coordination can include outcomes like errors in care, inability of patients and families to care for themselves, and untimely hospital readmissions. Definition and examination of care coordination activities in nursing practice assures that nurses will work to improve these kinds of outcomes by placing greater priority and consistency on their care coordination activities.

Another argument in favor of recognizing care coordination in everyday practice is the close relationship between clearly identifying what nurses do, being able to measure what they do, and being recognized for the value of this work. Recent studies demonstrate that nurses devote a considerable amount of time to coordinating care. Time and motion studies of hospital staff nurses by Hendrich, Chow, Skierczynski, and Lu (2008) found that these nurses spent almost one-fifth of their time communicating with other nurses and members of the healthcare team within and outside the hospital. Similarly, a recent examination of nurse and certified nursing assistant activities in nursing homes associated with reducing hospital admissions suggests that time spent in communication and transitional care activities also may be considerable (Lamb et al., 2011). Nursing's professional and leadership organizations, including the American Nurses Association (ANA, 2012) and the American Academy of Nursing (Cipriano, 2012) have drawn attention to the importance of nurse care coordination and have called for the development

Care coordination functions

Consider this definition of care coordination provided by the Agency for Health Care Research and Quality (McDonald et al., 2010, p. 4):

Care coordination is the deliberate organization of patient care activities between two or more participants (including the patient) involved in a patient's care to facilitate the appropriate delivery of health services. Organizing care includes marshaling of personnel and other resources needed to carry out all required patient care activities and is often managed by the exchange of information among participants responsible for different aspects of care.

List the ways you carry out these care coordination functions in your practice.

_____

_____

_____

of performance measures that capture this work and policy changes to support and reimburse it.

RECOGNIZING CARE COORDINATION IN YOUR PRACTICE

Many core nurse care coordination activities are identified, either implicitly or explicitly, in descriptions of care coordination models and programs. Take a moment to look at Table 2 in Chapter 4 (see page 65) that details common components of care coordination models. Regardless of whether we are talking about models from forty or more years ago, today's transitional care models, or patient-centered medical homes, care coordination entails a systematic set of activities including risk assessment, care planning, communication across providers and settings, and monitoring to assure that patients' needs are being met in a timely way. In the early years of managed care demonstrations and experiments, this was often referred to as making sure the patient received "the right care, at the right time, in the right place, at the right cost."

Taken one by one, each of these care coordination activities are recognizable in nursing practice. The following descriptions emphasize the features of care coordination activities to assist you in becoming more aware of when you are doing them. Examples are provided in the sidebar below.

You are coordinating care when...

Match each of the following activities to the description of care coordination activities in the narrative

- Work with patients and families to identify their goals and preferences
- Identify patients who do not have the needed skills or services to care for themselves
- Communicate with patients, families, and team members about the plan of care
- Get the needed people and services involved to keep the plan of care on track and timely
- Monitor that needed services have been identified, arranged, and delivered
- Assist patients and families to prepare a list of questions for upcoming visits with their primary care providers or specialists

Identifying Patients at Risk

One of the first steps in nursing care is to conduct a comprehensive assessment of the physical and social needs and issues patients are likely to confront in caring for themselves. Increasingly, we recognize constellations of problems and needs, such as multiple chronic conditions or lack of support systems or resources, which place individuals at risk for adverse quality outcomes. For instance, there is strong evidence that older individuals with multiple co-morbid conditions and a history of multiple hospital admissions are much more likely to be hospitalized again than older individuals who do not have these characteristics. They, like other at-risk populations, are very vulnerable to gaps in communication and care planning as they move across diverse providers and settings. Assessing risk, which all nurses do as soon as they meet and interact with patients and families, is foundational to all care coordination activities.

Communicating Accurate and Meaningful Patient-Centered Information

All patients, but particularly those at risk of poor outcomes, need extensive and often complicated relays of information between providers within a single setting and across settings. The relationship between care coordination, communication, and quality outcomes is detailed in upcoming chapters. As noted earlier, nurses typically are at the center of information exchanges in every modality possible: face-to-face, by telephone, by pager, by email, through telehealth, and, of course, through the health record. When nurses are referred to as the "hub" or "switchboard" of health care, the reference is to their vital work in assuring that the patient's needs and preferences are heard and integrated in the plan of care and that each person involved in the patient's care has the information needed to address them. The communication work that nurses do—and there is much of it—is core to effective care coordination. Coordination cannot happen without timely flow of accurate and meaningful information.

Managing the Plan of Care

What is the difference between having a plan of care that is simply a document that meets regulatory requirements and one that is a living, breathing tool to address patient needs and preferences? Translating the care plan into integrated action for patients, families, health professionals, and community programs is the central work of care coordination and where the work of nurses is most vital and likely to be the most invisible.

Consider the typical care plan in your practice. It likely includes the interplay of numerous providers and actions related to patient education, medication monitoring and management, diagnostic work-ups and follow-up, and referrals. You are doing care coordination each and every time you monitor how the plan of care is being implemented between and across providers, initiate activities to assure that the patient and his/her family's needs have been heard and incorporated, that the resources needed to activate the plan from insurance and transportation to availability of services are in place, and that the intended outcomes are achieved.

Preparing for Transitions

As patients and their families move from one provider to another or across settings, as they do at hospital discharge, it is a particularly vulnerable time for care to get fragmented and disorganized. In nursing, we often recognize this time as one in which patients can easily "fall through the cracks." Vital information may not be communicated and patients may not have the resources needed to take care of themselves or negotiate the leap from one setting to another. Metaphorically, they fall into the chasm between providers and settings. As a result, they may lose vital ground in their healing process, in their belief that they can care for themselves, and suffer preventable adverse events. Attention to these vulnerable transitions, referred to as transitional care, is a special area of emphasis within the broader domain of care coordination. We have learned that attending to this important time has significant payoffs in terms of reducing hospitalizations and medication errors, and improving the patient experience. In the sidebar on the next page, a foster parent describes the activities of a pediatric nurse who prepared her medically complex infant for transfer home.

In your practice, think about the actions you do to prepare patients and families for upcoming changes in providers and settings. In primary care, this could include helping them to identify and practice both clinical and care coordination questions they want to ask of the specialist to whom they're being referred. Coordination questions might include: "Do I need to see anyone else? Who will help me arrange that follow-up? What do you think about me seeing [blank]? Who will you communicate with about what we've talked about? My primary care provider (name)? The visiting nurse (name)? The physical therapist (name)? When will that happen?"

In home care, an obvious care coordination activity is helping facilitate communication and appointments with other care providers and community resources involved in their care. In addition, it may involve working with agency schedulers, patients, families, and other home care team members to organize home visits when the patient does not already have appointments away from home for a given day and to avoid multiple home care team visits on the same day. With good communication, team members scheduled

Preparing a medically complex infant and foster parent for hospital discharge

The discharge of my infant foster son was a very complex event. Due to health problems related to a premature birth, he required multiple medications and medical supplies as part of his daily care. Since he was coming into foster care, his discharge was complicated by the addition of social services involvement and a change in insurance coverage. After being in the hospital for many months, the decision to discharge by his surgeon was an unexpected and sudden determination, leaving only a short period of time for a large amount of coordination.

The staff nurse caring for my foster son coordinated every aspect of his discharge care. She worked with the surgical team to have all out-patient medications and supplies ordered through the correct agencies for delivery and ensured delivery prior to discharge. She worked with the hospital social worker and the child's caseworker to obtain all necessary legal paperwork for the hospital discharge to foster care. This RN worked closely with me to register and coordinate the child for developmental and medical services such as PT, OT, ST, and home nursing. In addition she educated me on his daily care and routines. She worked with the hospital's home nursing group to schedule teaching for me regarding the medical technology my foster son was being discharged with. She worked diligently with the child's new daycare center's nursing staff to teach them about his daily care, including his complex feeding schedule.

The RN made the child's discharge an easy transition despite a very complex and intricate set of needs and coordination. The child was able to be discharged in a short period of time with all aspects of his care already in place. The complicated care coordination that this RN completed resulted in the successful discharge of a medically fragile infant to a foster home in only a few days.

to visit can often address critical needs other team members have for information or observations related to health status.

In the hospital setting, there are often transitions in care between units. The patient monitoring activities of staff nurses create opportunities for improving the quality of those transitions through staff nurse care coordination (as illustrated in the sidebar on page 89). Hospitals also often have standardized sets of discharge planning activities to prepare patients and families for the transition out of the hospital to home, rehabilitation, assisted living, or long-term care. These activities may include self-care or parent education, medication review, care resources needed at home, or transfer of the plan of care to the receiving providers. If home care or other nurses will be involved in the transition and follow-up, it means communicating with them to facilitate a smooth care transition. However, it is critical to remember, as we talk about making nurse care coordination work visible, that there are many vital care coordination activities carried out by every nurse that works with a patient and family that set the stage for these specialized care coordination roles to be effective

Recognizing care coordination in your practice and in the practice of other nurses and professions requires defining the work and purposefully examining when and where it is happening. Once you start looking for care coordination work in nursing practice, you will see nurses assessing risk, facilitating communication, assuring that the plan of care is implemented, and facilitating transitions. It is important to "tune" your eyes and ears to how care coordination is embedded in everyday practice and how it relates to quality and safety outcomes.

At a system level, it is fairly straightforward to identify if mechanisms for these core care coordination functions are in place. For example, you could examine whether a hospital or a primary care center has a process and standardized tools in place to identify patients who are extremely vulnerable to gaps in care or are at risk of hospital admission or readmission. These tools are more common now as all organizations face incentives and penalties for hospital readmission. You also might look for whether there is a process in place to make sure that standardized patient information is shared between providers within and across settings.

THE VARIETY OF CARE COORDINATOR ROLES

In many settings, general care coordination activities carried out by staff nurses are supported and augmented by "nurse coordinators," APRNs, and other professionals, such as social workers, who occupy specialized care coordination or care management roles. Some of these roles have been present for some time or have come and gone in efforts to improve community-based care. More recently, widespread recognition of the importance of care coordination activities has led to the creation of many new roles designed specifically around care coordination responsibilities.

Care coordinators in specialized roles may work with high-risk children or adults over long periods of time or may focus primarily on transitions between settings. Typically, longer term care coordination is reserved for individuals with complex health and social needs who require extensive communication among providers and close integration of services. With the introduction of incentives for reducing avoidable hospitalization, there has been a substantial increase in the number and types of care coordination roles

> ## Monitoring as quality
>
> Dr. Judith Baggs and her colleagues demonstrated the importance of staff nurse monitoring and focused information exchange with the attending physician in determining a patient's readiness for discharge from the medical intensive care unit in two studies (Baggs, et al., 1992; Baggs et al., 1997; Baggs et al., 1999). They found that staff nurses' assessment of greater collaboration between the two team members related to the decision to discharge was associated with:
>
> * Lower mortality and readmission to the ICU
> * Greater satisfaction with the decision-making process
> * Greater satisfaction with the decision

focused on transitional care, such as health coaches and navigators. While many of the individuals in transitional care roles continue to be nurses, several new programs are exploring whether individuals from diverse professional, paraprofessional, and lay backgrounds can carry out selected care coordination activities. Expansions of the medical assistant role, for instance, are intended to fulfill some care coordination functions in the absence of nurses (Bodenheimer & Laing, 2007). Also, community health workers are being engaged to coordinate needs of disadvantaged and minority patients and populations to link them to appropriate and accessible care See the sidebar on the definition of community health workers on the next page.

Nurses providing general care in all settings need to understand how their "frontline" care coordination activities link with the care coordination activities of other more specialized care coordination roles, as well as with an interprofessional team of providers within and across care settings. Hand-offs between general and specialized care coordination functions are an important element of effective care for patients and families.

The proliferation of care coordination roles creates many new opportunities for nurses both within their current practices, and in new care delivery models. In addition to heightening awareness of care coordination in nursing practice, the academic community needs to assure that nurses are educated for care coordination. In *The Future of Nursing*, Virginia Tilden pointed out that curricula in care coordination are "underdeveloped" and that care coordination should be a cross-cutting strand throughout undergraduate and graduate nursing education (Tilden, 2010). In response, many schools of nursing are now incorporating content on the value of care coordination and care coordination competencies in their programs. Similarly, practice settings are providing on-site education for nurses to expand their care coordination functions. The following

> ### A definition of community health workers (CHWs)
>
> In Ohio, the Board of Nursing oversees program approval for the preparation of community health workers. Professional CHWs are organized as the Ohio Community Health Workers Association. They describe their role as:
>
> > "community representatives, [who] advocate for individuals and groups in the community by assisting them in accessing community health and supportive resources through the provision of education, role modeling, outreach, home visits, and referral services. ... [In order to eliminate disparities] community health workers provide a comprehensive link to community resources through family-based services focusing on success in health, education, and self-sufficiency." (Center for Healthy Communities, 2012)

section details the exciting efforts of a large primary care network to prepare staff nurses for new care coordination roles in patient-centered medical homes.

PREPARING NURSES FOR CARE COORDINATION IN THE PATIENT-CENTERED MEDICAL HOME

It is well-recognized that a central component of successful healthcare reform includes substantial redesign of our primary care system. The patient-centered medical home is an innovative primary care practice model that aims to improve patient and staff experiences, outcomes, safety, and efficiency in a manner consistent with current reform. The medical home rests on five conceptual pillars, including a patient-centered orientation, comprehensive team-based care, care coordination, easy access to care, and a systems-based approach to quality and safety. In addition, the model requires the use of health information technology to support proactive and population-based care as well as payment reform (AHRQ, 2011; Nutting, Crabtree, & McDaniel, 2012). As a vital member of the medical home interprofessional team, nurse care managers play a critical role in helping primary care practices function optimally.

The care manager role is relatively new in most primary care settings. Historically, many practices have tended to be hierarchical physician-centric systems where nurses have not practiced to the full extent of their licenses. Indeed, primary care nurses and other clinicians have often been "cast in unimaginative roles" (Nutting, Crabtree, & McDaniel, 2012, p. 2417). Thus, mentoring and supporting care managers in this new position requires more than an initial training program covering essential clinical content and role fundamentals. Opportunities for ongoing clinical supervision via case review and systematic opportunities for reflective practice are essential to successful enactment and full integration of the care manager role.

Many nurses in primary care settings are unaccustomed to taking time from their busy practice settings to review and reflect on their work with patients. Furthermore, they may conceptualize barriers to improved patient care simply as a function of clinician, staff, patient, and/or family personalities rather than systems' processes, which limits finding solutions and keeps nurses (and others) unclear about the nature of nurses' work (Ebright, 2004). To the extent that nurses define their care coordination activities as "just what we do," rather than recognizing such activities for the care processes they entail and the skill required to do them well, they minimize the central importance of their work to the team and the patients they serve. Providing a seasoned clinical mentor can be very helpful in supporting nurses' confidence and competence in identifying the essential care coordination components of risk assessment, communication of patient-centered information, as well as care plan and transition management. Once recognized as such, strategies for improving the quality and efficiency of delivering these components can be generated through collaborative learning discussions.

In Rochester, New York, care managers throughout a primary care network affiliated with a research intensive university meet monthly in small groups with a clinical nurse mentor. At the invitation of the network's medical director, the mentor initially collaborated in designing a training curriculum and delivering a portion of it for the inaugural group of nurse managers hired for the 23 patient-centered medical homes comprising the network. At the conclusion of the weeklong training program, the care managers expressed concern that they would struggle to refine and integrate the skills they had learned without additional coaching. The medical director, persuaded by the care managers' logic, negotiated and contracted with the mentor to develop and implement a process for continued education and training for the care managers. The mentor is an experienced leader with expertise in promoting motivational approaches to sustained behavior change, patient and family-centered care, team functioning, and systems navigation.

The purpose of the monthly meetings is for care managers to discuss challenges they face in working with patients, families, and colleagues to meet the goals of the medical home. Nurses rotate responsibility for patient and/or team case presentations, which then serve as focal points for small group discussion. Evidence from nursing, motivation science, and clinical practice guidelines for a variety of chronic illnesses, as well as the evidence available in collaboration, coordination, and teams, is applied to the "real life" practice scenarios provided by the case presentations. The *Monthly Care Manager Meetings* sidebar offers a typical case presentation.

The creativity and depth of the ideas generated through these small group discussions is enhanced by the considerable differences in how the 23 practices are organized and function. Often, a care manager in one practice has not even considered a strategy or intervention that another office has established simply because different practices have different norms, patient populations, and/or practice administrators. Processes for identifying and proactively reaching out to patients in need of preventive services such as mammography or colonoscopy, for example, may differ from practice to practice. Care managers often share efficient ways to collaborate with the data coordinators and physicians in their offices to ensure timely and careful attention to this key component of the medical home. It is not unusual for a care manager in one office to comment that a protocol in place in another office might be useful or "worth a try," or for the discussion to stimulate new ways of thinking about improving this important care process.

The care manager groups serve as learning collaboratives where non-judgmental self- and practice-reflection is valued, and where novel solutions to care coordination challenges are frequently generated. In the time between the monthly small group meetings, care managers and the clinical mentor also communicate online as needed. Additionally, the clinical mentor works with the care managers to identify common themes across the mentoring groups and, if the care managers are in agreement, shared issues are brought to the attention of the primary care network's senior leadership team so that improvements and policy changes can be made at the larger systems level.

There are two principles central to the success of this mentoring model. First, the approach is anchored in a general theory of motivation called self-determination theory, in which the care managers' psychological needs for autonomy, competence, and relatedness are honored and supported. The need for autonomy involves having a voice and feeling volitional about one's work. The need for competence refers to feeling confident that one has the capabilities, resources, and tools to do the work at hand while the need for relatedness is reflected by feeling emotionally connected with one's colleagues (Deci et al., 2001). There is evidence that, when employees' psychological needs are supported, they are more likely to adopt environmental regulations and norms (Lynch, Plant, & Ryan, 2005) Although more research is needed, this suggests that a need-supportive medical home work environment is more likely to employ and retain those who respect and abide by the central tenets of the medical home as evidenced by high quality coordinated care that is integrated, team-based, and patient-centered. Thus, the clinical mentor works with the nurses in ways that support their psychological needs. Autonomy

Monthly Care Manager Meetings

A care manager presented the significant challenges she and her team were facing in coordinating care with an elderly patient living with dementia, diabetes, and cardiovascular disease. The patient lived alone in her home with her 90-year-old frail husband who was doing his best to care for her. The patient was losing weight and was increasingly guarded and isolated. She was not taking her medications as prescribed. Repeated efforts to have the visiting nurse service intervene were unsuccessful as the patient would not permit the nurses access to her home. The care manager and the physician working with the patient were unable to reason with the patient who insisted "everything was fine." The initial care manager small group discussion focused on exploring patient–family–healthcare team role responsibilities, including identifying potential untapped resources. We strategized with the care manager about collaborating with the network social worker to convene a family meeting with the couple and their daughter who lived out of town along with the physician, social worker, and care manager. The meeting's purpose was to review the key issues and attempted solutions by all involved, and to develop a plan that would help ensure more consistent intervention and support. Since the family meeting, the patient has permitted visiting nurses into the home to assist with diabetes and medication management, and her daughter has been significantly more involved in her parents' day-to-day functioning. Collaboration between the couple's daughter and the medical home team has also improved.

support is provided by offering the nurses choices and options regarding ways of seeing or resolving challenges, as well as regarding issues for discussion. Competence support is strong because the mentor provides feedback in an informational way rather than in a judgmental or controlling manner. Also, support for relatedness is evident by the warm and caring interpersonal climate that characterizes the small group care manager meetings and online communications (Gagne & Deci, 2005).

The second principle is that the group discussions are confidential—not secretive, but confidential—in order to encourage openness and candor amongst the care managers as they discuss challenges to successful care coordination as well as other aspects of their roles. Specific practice issues are identified to senior network administrators only with approval from the care managers. For example, after the electronic medical record (EMR) was implemented throughout the network, the care managers were required to play a central role as "superusers." Many assessed that their central care coordination activities had become secondary as they were consumed with helping their practice partners use the EMR and assessing its impact on workflow. The loss of this central function disturbed the nurses greatly and threatened the viability of their roles. Thus, in collaboration with the clinical mentor, senior administrative network leaders were informed of the nurses' observations and concerns. An intervention was designed that assisted the care managers in collectively identifying and discussing their central care collaborative coordination responsibilities and other key aspects of their role before implementation of the EMR. The intervention helped reorient the nurses to their primary responsibilities, while providing senior administrators with important feedback about the potential threats to the care coordination activities upon which the success of the medical home largely rests. The mentoring model, which has been in place for nearly two years, has been very well received by the nurse care managers and primary care network administrators.

The primary care medical home model continues to develop and expand throughout the nation's healthcare system. Given the pivotal role of nurse care managers on teams charged with ensuring well-coordinated, patient-centered care for those served by the medical home, it is essential to assist nurses in reflecting systematically on their practice in this evolving model. The clinical mentoring approach described in this chapter constitutes one system's approach to cultivating such reflective practice. Experience to date suggests that it has been a prudent investment in supporting primary care practice improvement.

CONCLUSION

Care coordination continues to be a major strength and contribution of the nursing profession to the overall quality and safety of our healthcare system. In this chapter, we have made the case for heightening the visibility and understanding of care coordination activities in all nursing roles and practice settings. Recognizing care coordination in both general and specialized nursing roles is essential for advancing this work and assuring that quality and cost goals are met. Both the education and practice communities play important roles in assuring that nurses are prepared to perform effective care coordination and to capitalize on new opportunities.

REFERENCES

Agency for Healthcare Research and Quality (AHRQ). (2011). What is the PCMH? AHRQ's definition of the medical home. Retrieved from http://pcmh.ahrq.gov/portal/server.pt/community/pcmh__home/1483/what_is_pcmh_

American Nurses Association (ANA). (2012). *Position statement: Care coordination and registered nurses' essential role*. Retrieved from http://www.nursingworld.org/position/care-coordination.aspx

Baggs, J. G., Ryan, S. A., Phelps, C. E. Richeson J. F., & Johnson, J. E. (1992). The association between interdisciplinary collaboration and patient outcomes in medical intensive care. *Heart & Lung, 21*, 18–24.

Baggs, J. G., Schmitt, M. H., Mushlin, A. I., Eldredge, D. H., Oakes, D., & Hutson, A. D. (1997). Nurse–physician collaboration and satisfaction with the decision making process in three critical care units. *American Journal of Critical Care, 6*, 393–399.

Baggs, J. G., Schmitt, M. H., Mushlin, A. I., Mitchell, P. H., Eldredge, D. H., Oakes, D., et al. (1999). Association between nurse–physician collaboration and patient outcomes in three intensive care units. *Critical Care Medicine, 27*, 1991–1998.

Bodenheimer, T., & Laing, B. Y. (2007). The teamled model of primary care. *Annals of Family Medicine, 5*(5), 457–461.

Brown, R. S., Peikes, D., Peterson, G., Shore, J., & Razafindrakoto, C. M. (2012). Six features of Medicare Coordinated Care Demonstration programs that cut hospital admissions of high risk patients. *Health Affairs, 31*(3) 1156–1167.

Center for Healthy Communities. (2012). What are community health workers? Retrieved from http://www.med.wright.edu/chc/programs/ochwa

Centers for Medicare and Medicaid Services (CMS). (2013). Accountable care organizations. Retrieved from http://www.cms.gov/Medicare/Medicare-Fee-for-Service-Payment/ACO/index.html

Cipriano, P. (2012). The imperative for patient, family, and population-centered interprofessional approaches to care coordination and transitional care: A policy brief by the American Academy of Nursing's Care Coordination Task Force. *Nursing Outlook, 60* (5), 330–333.

Deci, E. L., Ryan, R. M., Gagné, M., Leone, D. R., Usunov, J., & Kornazheva, B. P. (2001). Need satisfaction, motivation, and well-being in the work organizations of a former Eastern Bloc country. *Personality and Social Psychology Bulletin, 27*, 930–942.

Ebright, P. R. (2004). Understanding nurse work. *Clinical Nurse Specialist, 18*, 168–170.

Gagne, M., & Deci, E. (2005). Self-determination theory and work motivation. *Journal of Organizational Behavior, 26*, 331–362.

Gürses, A. P., Carayon, P., & Wall, M. (2009). Impact of performance obstacles on intensive care nurses' workload, perceived quality and safety of care, and quality of working life. *Health Services Research, 44*(2 Part I), 422–443.

Hendrich, A., Chow, M., Skierczynski, R. A., Lu, Z. (2008). A 36-hospital time and motion study: How do medical surgical nurses spend their time? *The Permanente Journal, 12*(3), 25–34.

Institute for Health Care Improvement (IHI). (2013). The IHI Triple Aim. Retrieved from http://www.ihi.org/offerings/Initiatives/TripleAim/Pages/default.aspx

Institute of Medicine (IOM). (2003). *Priority areas for national action: Transforming health care quality*. Washington, DC: The National Academies Press.

Institute of Medicine (IOM). (2010). *The future of nursing: Leading change, advancing health*. Washington, DC: The National Academies Press.

Lamb, G., Tappen, R., Diaz, S., Herndon, L., Ouslander, J. (2011). Avoidability of hospital transfers of nursing home residents: Perspectives of front-line staff. *Journal of the American Geriatrics* Society, *59,* 1665–1672.

Lynch, M. F., Plant, R. W., & Ryan, R. M. (2005). Psychological needs and threat to safety: Implications for staff and patients in a psychiatric hospital for youth. *Professional Psychology, 36,* 415–425.

McDonald, K. M., Schultz, E., Albin, L., Pineda, N., Lonhard, J., Sundaram, C., Smith-Spangler, C., Brustrom, J., & Malcolm, E. (2010). *Care coordination atlas version 3* (Prepared by Stanford University under subcontract to Battelle on Contract No. 290-04-0020). AHRQ Publication No: 11-0023-EF. Rockville, MD: Agency for Research and Quality.

National Committee for Quality Assurance. (2011). NCQA Patient-centered medical home. Retrieved from http://www.ncqa.org/portals/0/PCMH%20brochure-web.pdf

National Quality Forum (NQF). (2010). *Preferred practices and performance measures for measuring and reporting care coordination: A consensus report.* Washington, DC:NQF.

Nutting, P. A., Crabtree, B. F., & McDaniel, R. R. (2012). Small primary care practices face four hurdles—including a physician-centric mind-set—in becoming medical homes. *Health Affairs, 31,* 2417–2422. doi: 10.1377/hlthadd.2011.0974

Tilden, V. (2010). The future of nursing education. In Institute of Medicine, *The future of nursing*, Appendix 1, (pp. 551–564). Washington, DC: The National Academies Press.

Chapter 6

The Role of Nursing Leaders in Advancing Care Coordination

Ingrid Duva, PhD, RN

T he United States has set forth ambitious goals for healthcare reform. Achieving better health at a more reasonable cost requires close attention to the systems and resources supporting effective practice. The role of leaders in health systems is to create a shared vision for goal achievement, build supportive environments, and develop the capability of staff and colleagues to practice effectively and to their fullest capacity (IOM, 2010). Nurse leaders play a critical role promoting the unique and valuable contributions of nursing to health system transformation. The previous chapter addressed the importance of defining, recognizing, and improving the work of care coordination in all practice settings. Effective care coordination is essential to meet the promise of accessible, high quality, affordable care for all Americans. Similarly, effective nurse leadership is critical so that nurses can perform these vital care coordination activities to have the desired impact on patient care and system outcomes. This chapter examines the role of nursing leadership in care coordination. Leadership strategies and models best aligned to advancing care coordination are emphasized.

NURSE LEADERSHIP MAKES A DIFFERENCE

The need for leaders capable of driving the organizational and system changes necessary to meet the goals of healthcare reform goes without saying. Additionally, strong nursing leadership is clearly needed to accelerate nurse care coordination for patients within these organizations, health systems, and throughout the community. Core leadership competencies (see Figure 1), such as those defined as critical for executive leaders by Ibarra & Obodaru (2009), are vital to embedding and sustaining good care coordination practices in all healthcare settings. All care coordination models rely on the effective communication and teamwork reflected by these competencies, as well as shared vision and staff engagement for needed system changes and improvement.

Better outcomes, including patient and nurse outcomes, are linked to strong nurse leadership. A systematic review by Wong and Cummings (2007) demonstrated evidence of significant associations between nurse leadership and the following patient care outcomes: satisfaction, mortality, morbidity, adverse events, and complications (Wong & Cummings, 2007). The studies used varying measures and identified a variety of leadership attributes. However, the improved patient outcomes were all linked to the leaders with behaviors consistently rated higher by nurses in all studies. The common behaviors are consistent with the leadership competencies identified in Figure 1. They have a relational orientation, set a vision for the future, and communicate clear expectations for nurse performance (Wong & Cummings, 2007). Emerging studies of leadership build on these findings. Effective leadership behaviors are more interactive and focus on relationships. These behaviors can facilitate change and are consistent with a "transformational" leadership style.

TRANSFORMATIONAL LEADERSHIP SUPPORTS IMPROVEMENT

Transformational leadership styles can benefit leaders striving for broad organizational and cultural change and are promoted to reach the goals of reform. An increased commitment to change initiatives, which is critical to sustaining improvement, is achieved with this leadership style (Herold, Fedor, Caldwell, & Liu, 2008). The principles of transformational leadership (see Figure 2) are recognized as standard for today's executive nurse leaders (ANA, 2010; AONE, 2005).

Achieving transformational leadership, as suggested by leading scholar James Burns, depends on the quality of the leader–follower interactions (2003). Both the leader and the follower have the ability to raise each other to a higher level of motivation for work and achievement. In contrast, the transactional leader relies on task management as a means to achieve the goals of day-to-day work. The transformational leader needs to incorporate traditional management practices consistent with transactional leadership to be successful. Additionally, the successful transformational leader goes beyond task orientation to empower followers to reach toward greater goals (Burns, 2003). This can move a team, organization, or system to greater accomplishments. The contributions of both the leader and the follower are equally important in transformational leadership. Momentum for change, particularly the large scale change that is needed to redefine traditional processes, inefficient systems, and ineffective roles and relationships, has to be well-established and sustainable. Executive nurse leaders (and nurses performing other

1. Empowering by delegating and sharing information

2. Energizing and motivating employees

3. Designing systems to align employee behavior to organizational goals and values

4. Rewarding and giving constructive feedback

5. Teambuilding, promoting collaboration, and encouraging constructive feedback

6. Making employees aware of outside constituencies

7. Instilling a global mindset to address cultural differences represented in the organization

8. Encouraging tenacity and courage through personal example

9. Fostering trust in the organization by creating an emotionally intelligent workforce

10. Envisioning

(Source: Adapted from Ibarra & Obodaru, 2009)

Figure 1 Executive Leadership Competencies

high-level leadership roles) have the ability to be transformative and, to lead change, it must be harnessed to realize improvements and sustain the seamless care coordination called for in reform.

NURSES HAVE "THE RIGHT STUFF" TO ADVANCE CARE COORDINATION

We have a strong foundation for nurse executives and other levels of nursing leadership to advance nurse care coordination and deliver on the goals of reform. Practical experience as direct and indirect caregivers across a broad spectrum of settings provides coordination expertise. Nurses' great experiential knowledge at the point of care affords an understanding of the needs of the patients and the nuances of the system in which the care is provided. This knowledge is invaluable as our system absorbs change and adapts to economic demands. Higher relational and communication skills are promoted as part of the transformational leadership style. Additionally, the leadership training provided in nursing includes the requisite competencies called for by other health professional programs to lead in the healthcare system. In fact, the American Organization of Nurse

Transactional Leader	Transformational Leader
Task management orientation	Common value orientation
Takes care of people and problems	Commits to people and problem solving
Bargains to meet goals	Inspires shared goals
Communicates current values	Communicates long-term values
Examines cause of problems	Evaluates effects of problems
Rewards are contingent	Invests in people

(*Source:* Adapted from Burns, 2003)

Figure 2 Comparison of Leadership Styles

Executives (AONE) requires equivalent, if not more, training for effective leadership skills than the general healthcare executive (HCLE) or the physician executive (ACMPE) and have comparable expectations in leadership roles (Vandriel, Bellack, & O'Neil, 2012).

Nurse presence at the top levels of leadership in healthcare is growing. Nurse CEOs, considered the highest leadership position in an organization, have increased by almost 10% since 2004 and when surveyed, 19% of chief nurses aspired to be a chief executive officer (Falter, 2012). Healthcare organizations are becoming more complex and larger, merging vertically and horizontally, and treating more types of patients in new and innovative settings. The opportunities for nurses to hold executive positions are also broadening, and go beyond governance of nursing and beyond single settings. This represents a great opportunity. These high-level leaders influence the priorities for patient care and, therefore, are critical champions for care coordination.

Positional power accompanies formal, especially high level, leadership positions and facilitates leadership effectiveness. It represents the additional authority and accountability that accompanies formal leadership roles and increases with the level of leadership. Positional power can increase the opportunity to drive the future direction for nurse care coordination. For example, it facilitates understanding of the critical role of the nurse as the coordinator of care, the opportunity for nurses leading interprofessional teams to coordinate care, and the designing of roles for team-based provision of care coordination. Yet, an effective leadership style, such as transformational leadership, for any level leader can still strengthen the platform for nursing and facilitate overall care coordination goals. Nurse leaders at all levels can identify the contributions of nurses, prioritize care coordination processes, and thoughtfully allocate resources to facilitate this work. In addition, it is important that nurse leaders at all levels provide visible and vocal support for care coordination and the work nurses are doing.

LEADING FROM WITHIN: THE PRACTICE OF NURSE CARE COORDINATION

Nurses are positioned in every sector of health care to provide leadership to advance and improve care coordination. Nurses at the point of care, in specialized care coordination roles, in management, and in formal leadership positions all have the opportunity to bring attention to fundamental care coordination activities performed by nurses. As described in the previous chapter, care coordination is a core nursing process. Nurses in all settings perform risk assessments, communicate across settings, collaborate with fellow team members, participate in care planning with patients and family members, and plan for a smooth discharge. Nurse care coordination transcends settings. For example, nurses can be assigned to oversee patient transitions from the hospital to home or long-term care. Rehabilitation and sub-acute care nurses often plan for care longitudinally, connecting chronically ill or functionally limited patients to community resources according to their ongoing needs (Marek, Popejoy, Petroski, & Rantz, 2006; Naylor et al., 2004; Rastkar, Zweig, Delzell, & Davis, 2002; Rogers, 2008; Skillings & MacLeod, 2009).

Nursing's historical orientation to patient-centered and population-based care, both of which are being rediscovered at an amazing pace, also provides significant cache for front-line staff to lead the development of new and improved care coordination programs. Patient-centered care coordination, now a core professional standard and competency for all nurses (ANA, 2012), should be the foundation for all care coordination programs. Within their teams, including patients and families, nurses can foster the use of evidence-based guidelines for addressing the needs and preferences of patients and families in both the development and communication of the plan of care. Core elements of population-based care, such as risk assessment and customized risk-based interventions, are also central to all care coordination programs. These are expected skill sets and competencies that all nurses can bring to their organization's efforts to improve care coordination and patient outcomes. These include initiatives to reduce avoidable hospitalizations, and improve the use of community-based resources and the quality of the patient experience regardless of setting.

Nurses in specialized care coordination roles, such as case managers, discharge planners and coaches, have unique leadership opportunities. As the most visible practitioners of care coordination, they can assist front-line staff to make their diverse care coordination activities more visible in system change initiatives. Nurse case managers and discharge planners play a vital part in expanding thinking about integration of services across the continuum of care, not just between hospital and home. In the evolution of care coordination models, they serve as an important bridge between an outdated hospital-centric system and new, more integrated systems that include prevention, promotion, and self-care management in an array of community settings. Together with front-line staff and members of the interprofessional healthcare team, their work is focused toward achievement of seamless, integrated care with less duplication and fragmentation. The nursing profession should recognize and capitalize on nurses in emerging care coordination roles as change-agents and leaders with their interprofessional teams, health systems, and communities.

Advanced practice nurses (APRNs) also have special opportunities to advance care coordination. In their roles as primary care providers and advanced practitioners in numerous clinical domains, such as intensive care, women's health, behavioral health, and other settings, APRNs perform and oversee care coordination. APRNs often identify the gaps in the continuity of care and are positioned to lead improvement efforts both within their care team and system-wide. Typically, the APRN works closely with physicians or specialists, pharmacists, and social workers, as well as nurse members of their team. Nurses in provider or advance practice roles can serve as a conduit for communication among these groups of professionals serving different roles on the team. Often these individuals practice in a shared location but may still function in siloes. The APRN has an opportunity to be a bridge builder and champion for new models that can enhance communication and continuity of care. The APRN also can educate nurse team members about care coordination and model salient care coordination activities that improve patient outcomes.

MOVING NURSE CARE COORDINATION AHEAD IN THE GAME

Together, point-of-care nurses and nurse leaders have created a solid groundwork for moving care coordination into the future. Nursing education programs need to incorporate evolving competencies to assure nurses have the right skills to continue to lead in dynamic health systems (see Figure 3). According to Huston (2008), these skills are responsive to the current and future challenges in health care which will still rely on care coordination as a pivotal strategy. These skills are strikingly similar to the executive leadership competencies for great leaders identified by Ibarra and Obodaru (2009).

Engaging all nurses in the effort to improve and advance care coordination is important; however, engaging the highest levels of leadership (e.g., chief nursing officers, regional or patient care directors) is essential. Focusing the top nursing leadership on three key areas can put nurse care coordination on the fast-track so that it can be "a game changer" for health care. Drawing from organizational, leadership, and improvement literature to create and communicate a shared vision, providing a supportive work

1. A global perspective or mindset regarding healthcare and professional nursing issues

2. Technology skills which facilitate mobility and portability of relationships, interactions, and operational processes

3. Expert decision-making skills rooted in empirical science

4. The ability to create organization cultures that permeate quality healthcare and patient/worker safety

5. Understanding and appropriately intervening in political processes

6. Highly developed collaborative and team building skills

7. The ability to balance authenticity and performance expectations

8. Being able to envision and proactively adapt to a healthcare system characterized by rapid change and chaos

(Source: Huston, 2008).

Figure 3 Eight Essential Nurse Leader Competencies for 2020

environment, and building personal and professional expertise are the keys to advancing and improving this critical work (Falter, 2012; Ibarra & Obodaru, 2009; Lukas et al., 2007; Ogrinc et al., 2012). Each of these three central leadership functions is described below.

CREATING AND COMMUNICATING A SHARED VISION

First, nurse leaders need to create a shared vision for care coordination and align goals for nursing. Vision is critical in this dynamic environment. Ibarra and Obodaru (2009) went so far as to suggest that envisioning might be the single most important skill for leadership effectiveness. Lacking a clear priority for care coordination or lack of clarity about what care coordination is will undermine nursing performance. Setting a vision for the organization, system, or community motivates and provides momentum to reach goals. A vision articulates clearly a new and better future state. It integrates the needs of both the larger and the local context. Successful leaders not only create a vision, but they can communicate the vision to others, even breaking it down into smaller, achievable steps for more immediate and gratifying success.

The vision for care coordination is to pave the way to improved health care for the future encompassing the trifecta of increased access, improved quality, and decreased cost. An appropriate vision integrates with organization, system, and individual priorities. For nurse care coordination, a common vision is to position nurses within interprofessional teams to perform this core nursing process and contribute to better patient outcomes. By doing so, nurses will play a major part in shifting healthcare outcomes for the better. Said another way, health care is being reformed, but ultimately nurse care coordination will be the difference. This vision must be communicated by leaders.

Goals for the stakeholders should also align. When goals do not align, it is the leader's responsibility to assist staff and members of the interprofessional team to find ways to bring them together. For example, some patients and their family members may prefer for the patient to remain in the hospital for a longer stay than medically necessary. The system goal is likely to discharge the patient as soon as he or she is medically stable. In this situation, the leader may need to step in and assist with the development of a plan that helps the patient and family feel comfortable with the care transition and, at the same time, uses both patient and hospital resources effectively and efficiently.

DEVELOPING SUPPORTIVE WORK ENVIRONMENTS

Keeping Patients Safe (IOM, 2004), the same report that recognized the critical role of nurses in care coordination, urged attention to the work environment to promote patient safety. The experts compiling this report collected evidence showing that many nurses' work environments were characterized by threats to patient safety such as poor management practices, insufficient staffing patterns, and poor work design and organizational culture. Supportive work environments, on the other hand, can facilitate nurse care coordination and remove barriers to this critical work.

The nurses' work environment is defined as "the organizational characteristics of a work setting that facilitate or constrain professional nursing practice" and contribute to an empowered nursing practice (Lake, 2002; Pearson et al., 2006). Essentially, it is part of the broad infrastructure that needs to be in place so that nurse care coordination can occur. This infrastructure will consist of a work environment to support care coordination, and should include the presence of supportive systems, processes, and structures (see the sidebar on the next page). Time, training, and equipment are examples of resources that support care coordination. These resources are components of the systems, processes, and structures that need to be present and set the context for care coordination.

Effective leaders create supportive work environments that facilitate professional nursing practice. Not only are these work environments associated with higher nurse satisfaction and reduced nursing turnover, but also with better patient outcomes (Aiken, Clarke, & Sloane, 2008; Aiken, Smith, & Lake, 1994; Estabrooks, Midodzki, Cummings,

Technology Support for Nurse Care Coordination Practice

An RN applies population health management strategies in her care coordination role as a primary care nurse care manager. In the past, the nurse had to find each person with diabetes through a record review and create a manual system for tracking appointments. Now, the nurse uses an automated system that flags all patients with a diagnosis of diabetes for regular primary care visits and quarterly laboratory appointments for hemoglobin A1C testing. Rather than spend time searching for patient information, the nurse concentrates on analyzing the information and working with patients and members of the care team to develop an effective care plan.

Consider how implementation of the electronic health record contributes to system, structural, and processes changes that support effective care coordination.

Ricker, & Giovenetti, 2005; Friese, 2005, 2008). The supportive work environment provides the context for nursing work, which, in turn, supports the work itself: nurse care coordination. Preliminary evidence exists to support this relationship. In one study, a higher level of professional practice and team functioning in the work environment was associated with less time being spent on care coordination according to their level of prioritization. The data also showed that nurses perceiving a higher level professional practice environment and higher team functioning spent less time on and less frequently performed activities considered duplicative, such as backfilling work for others, or following up with other professionals regarding omitted tasks (Duva, 2010). Thus, a positive work environment can support care coordination, which ultimately can lead to better patient outcomes.

Examining the link between work environments and nursing practice is not new. Much of this work began in the early 1980s with the study of Magnet™ hospitals. These organizations were coined Magnet hospitals because they had higher recruitment and retention during a time of a severe nursing shortage. Studies found these "magnetic hospitals" had common organizational characteristics: autonomy, control over practice, positive nurse–physician relationships, and access to resources. Nurses were more attracted to working in these hospitals than nearby competitor hospitals. Subsequently, these hospitals were also found to have better patient outcomes. Patient satisfaction was higher and patient morbidity and mortality was lower (Aiken et al., 2008; Aiken et al., 1994; Estabrooks et al., 2005; Friese, 2008).

Over time, the identification of better outcomes at Magnet™ hospitals led to the categorization of 14 Forces of Magnetism. These are organizational characteristics essential to support nursing excellence (ANCC, 2013a). The more current Magnet Model (ANCC, 2013b) reflects important mutually interacting system, structural, and process forces which are expressed in terms of organizational qualities: structural empowerment; new knowledge, improvements, and innovations; exemplary professional practice, transformational leadership; empirical outcomes and their relationship to the global healthcare environment and improved outcomes. This model can apply to any environment where professional nurses are working. The crux of the model is that it provides structural support for professional practice. The organization and workplace enable exemplary practice and innovation. In these environments, nurses take accountability for excellent practice. They engage in evidence-based care coordination practices, such as involving the family when planning for the patients' home care needs to be met. They use new knowledge and innovative approaches, such as the team approach to care advocated for in patient-centered medical care homes. The result is measurable outcomes that demonstrate continued excellence, such as reducing unnecessary readmissions or expediting an appointment by improving the accuracy of communication between the specialist and the primary care provider.

In recent literature, effective work environments are referred to as "healthy work environments" (Kramer & Schmalenberg, 2010). Building on the Magnet research are the American Association of Critical Care Nurses (AACN) standards, which state that healthy work environments optimize the relationship among leadership, empowerment, innovation, and exemplary professional practice (Huston, 2008). In these environments, "leaders provide the practices, systems, and policies that enable clinical nurses to engage in the work essential to safe and quality patient care" (Kramer, Schmalenberg, & Maguire, 2010 p.1). A meta-analysis of the existing study of nurse work environments resulted in a composite of nine best leadership practices and structures (see Figure 4) (Kramer & Schmalenberg, 2010). Note the similarities between the structural characteristics in this list and the previously described Magnet model, as well as the similarity between the leadership competencies to the competencies for leadership listed earlier in this chapter (see Figures 1 and 3).

As a model for supporting excellent nursing, the "essentials" for a healthy work environment offers another approach to advance nurse care coordination. The focus shifts from just "having the right things" in place to "doing the right things" so that better outcomes are achieved (Kramer, Schmalenberg, & McGuire, 2010,). Kramer & Schmalenberg (2008) contend that this is a more direct and effective approach to

1. Quality leadership at all levels in the organization

2. Availability of and support for education, career, performance, and competence development

3. Administrative sanction for autonomous and collaborative practice

4. Evidence-based practice education and operational supports

5. Culture, practice, and opportunity to learn interdisciplinary collaboration

6. Empowered, shared decision-making structures for control of the context of nursing practice

7. Generation and nurturance of a patient-centered culture

8. Staffing structures that take into account RN competence, patient acuity, and teamwork

9. Development and support of intradisciplinary teamwork

(Source: Kramer & Schmalenberg, 2010; p. 10)

Figure 4 Nine Structures/Best Leadership Practices
Essential for Healthy Work Environments

improving outcomes. Accordingly, nurse leaders who assess and measure the extent to which the right structures and processes are present will be more successful improving nurse care coordination.

Nurse leaders can expect to create and refine healthy work environments in the midst of significant change in the healthcare system, including the widespread use of health information technology. Their strategies for supporting care coordination will need to be matched to the priorities and workforce capacity in each practice setting. It is likely that new practice arrangements, such as accountable care organizations or patient-centered medical homes, will require different structures and processes for care coordination. Leaders need to be responsive to these changes and evaluate their impact on nursing practice and outcomes.

BUILDING EXPERTISE: SYSTEM'S THINKING AND TEAMWORK

The ability to communicate and engender systems thinking across all providers is essential for the development and advancement of integrative work like care coordination. William Deming, one of the foremost leaders in quality improvement, defined a system as a network of interdependent components that work together to accomplish a specific aim (Nelson, Batalden, and Godfrey, 2007). Each part of a system must work together to achieve its goals. In health care, care coordination is foundational to assuring that all parts of the system communicate with each other and contribute to one unified plan of care for each patient.

Much of the current leadership thinking and research is grounded in systems models and frameworks. Donabedian's framework linking organizational structures, processes, and outcomes (see Figure 5), for example, has been guiding the evaluation and improvement of medical care and healthcare systems for over 40 years. This framework also provided the foundation for the early studies leading to the Magnet Recognition Program Model and the Essentials for a Healthy Work Environment described previously. It is readily applicable to the kind of thinking and leadership needed to improve care coordination in any setting and is consistent with the range and type of leadership strategies discussed earlier.

Nursing leaders also have an important role in building a culture of teamwork and collaboration (see the sidebar on the next page). Opportunities to advance care coordination models and lead system change are tied to effective team performance (AACN, 2008). Many healthcare organizations have embarked on extensive teamwork train-

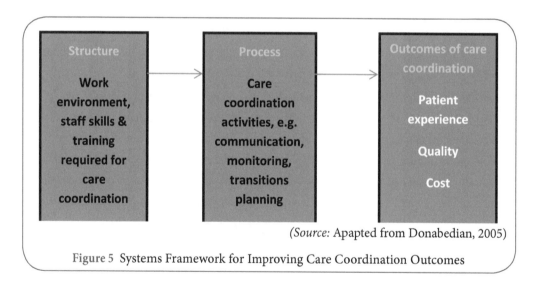

(Source: Apapted from Donabedian, 2005)

Figure 5 Systems Framework for Improving Care Coordination Outcomes

ing programs for staff members. The TeamSTEPPS (Strategies and Tools to Enhance Performance and Patient Safety) program, for example, provides a model for developing and improving teamwork (TeamSTEPPS, n.d.). The TeamSTEPPS toolkit includes

> ## Care Coordination, Collaboration, and Teamwork
>
> You practice as an APRN in a primary care clinic that is part of a large primary care network. Each of the clinics in the network has embraced the concept of team practice and is experimenting with teams composed of primary care providers, registered nurses, and medical assistants supported by front office and clerical staff. As team leader, you have the opportunity to enable the full scope of practice of each team member and to create an environment for optimal team performance. The registered nurses on your team believe they can make significant contributions to patient care by focusing on and expanding their care coordination functions.
>
> What strategies would you use to support the RNs on your team to improve and expand their care coordination activities?
>
> How would you assist them to demonstrate their contribution to team performance?

surveys and observational tools that staff can be encouraged to incorporate in efforts to improve collaborative performance. Other tools focus specifically on teamwork behaviors such as relational coordination that are necessary for care coordination are becoming available (Gittell, n.d., 2002a, 2002b, 2007; Gittell et. al., 2000; OPM.gov, n.d.).

CONCLUSION

Nursing leadership is needed to assure the spread and uptake of innovative and effective care coordination across the continuum of care. The context in which nurses provide care coordination will undoubtedly evolve to keep pace with the rapid changes in patient-care needs and our healthcare system. New work environments will emerge to meet the needs of our more fluid and mobile patterns of work and life. However, the foundation is in place for nurses to continue to make meaningful contributions to patient care coordination despite changing work environments. The models for supportive work environments discussed in this chapter all rely on flexible systems thinking and guide leadership practices relevant to supporting care coordination in all practice settings. Systems thinking and structural work enhancements will improve nursing capacity to perform care coordination within and across settings. Leadership is vital to energize and empower nurses and members of the healthcare team to embrace the changes ahead.

REFERENCES

Aiken, L. H., Clarke, S. P., & Sloane, D. M. (2008). Effects of hospital care environment on patient mortality and nurse outcomes. *Journal of Nursing Administration, 38*(5), 223–229.

Aiken, L. H., Smith, H. L., & Lake, E. T. (1994). Lower Medicare mortality among a set of hospitals known for good nursing care. *Medical Care,* 771–787.

American Nurses Association. (ANA). (2010). *Nursing administration: Scope and standards of practice.* Silver Spring, MD: Nursesbooks.org.

American Nurses Credentialing Center (ANCC) (2013a). Forces of Magnetism. Retrieved from http://www.nursecredentialing.org/ForcesofMagnetism.asp

American Nurses Credentialing Center (ANCC) (2013b). Magnet Recognition Program® Model. Retrieved from www.nursecredentialing.org/Magnet/ProgramOverview/New-Magnet-Model

American Organization of Nurse Executives (AONE). (2005). Nurse executive competencies. *Nurse Leader, 3,* 50–56.

Burns, J. M. (2003). *Transformational Leadership.* New York, NY: Grove/Atlantic, Inc.

Donabedian, Avedis (2005). Evaluating the quality of medical care. *The Milbank Quarterly 83*(4): 691–729.

Duva, I. H. (2010). *Factors impacting staff nurse care coordination.* (PhD thesis), Emory University, Atlanta, GA.

Estabrooks, C. A., Midodzki, W. K., Cummings, G. G., Ricker, K. L., & Giovenetti, P. (2005). The impact of hospital nursing characteristics on 30-day mortality. *Nursing Research, 54*(2), 74–84.

Falter, E. (2012). Nursing leadership…From the board room to the bedside. *Nursing Administration Quarterly, 36*(1), 17–23.

Friese, C. R. (2005). Nurse practice environments and outcomes: Implications for oncology nursing. *Oncology Nursing Forum, 32*(4), 765–772.

Friese, C. R. (2008). Hospital nurse practice environments and outcomes for surgical oncology patients. *Health Services Research, 43*(4), 1145–1163.

Gittell, J. H. (2002a). Coordinating mechanisms in care provider groups: Relational coordination as a mediator and input uncertainty as a moderator of performance effects. *Management Science, 48*(11), 1408–1426.

Gittell, J. H. (2002b). Relationships between service providers and their impact on customers. *Journal of Service Research, 4*(4), 299–311.

Gittell, J. H. (2007). *Relational coordination: Recommendations for theory, measurement and analysis.* Brandeis University. Waltham, MA.

Gittell, J. H. (n.d.). Measuring relational coordination. Retrieved from http://rcrc.brandeis.edu/survey/measuring.html

Gittell, J. H., Fairfield, K. M., Bierbaum, B., Head, W., Jackson, R., Kelly, M., … Zuckerman, J. (2000). Impact of relational coordination on quality of care, postoperative pain and functioning, and length of stay: a nine-hospital study of surgical patients. *Medical Care, 38*(8), 807–819.

Herold, D. M., Fedor, D. B., Caldwell, S., & Liu, Y. (2008). The effects of transformational and change leadership on employees' commitment to change: A multilevel study. *Journal of Applied Pyschology, 93*(2), 346–357.

Huston, C. J. (2008). Preparing nurse leaders for 2020. *Journal of Nursing Management, 16*, 905–911.

Ibarra, H., & Obodaru, O. (2009). Women and the vision thing. *Harvard Business Review*, 62–70.

Institute of Medicine (IOM). (2010). *The future of nursing: Leading change, advancing health.* Washington, DC: National Academies Press.

Institute of Medicine (IOM). 2004.*Keeping patientssafe: Transforming the work environment of nurses.* Washington, DC: National Academies Press.

Kramer, M., Schmalenberg, C., & McGuire, P. (2010). Nine structures and leadership practices essential for of healthy (magnetic) work environments. *Nursing Administration Quarterly, 34*(1), 4–17.

Lake, E. T. (2002). Development of the practice environment scale of the nursing work index. *Research in Nursing and Health, 25*, 176–188

Lukas, C. V., Holmes, S. K., Cohen, A. B., Restuccia, J., Cramer, I. E., Shwartz, M., & Charns, M.P. (2007). An organizational model of transformational change in healthcare systems. *Health Care Management Review, 32*(4), 309–320.

Marek, K. D., Popejoy, L., Petroski, G., & Rantz, M. (2006). Nurse care coordination in community-based long-term care. *Journal of Nursing Scholarship, 38*(1), 80–86.

Naylor, M. D., Brooten, D. A., Campbell, R. L., Maislin, G., McCauley, K. M., & Schwartz, J. S. (2004). Transitional care of older adults hospitalized with heart failure: A randomized, controlled trial. *Journal of the American Geriatric Society, 52*(5), 675–684.

Ogrinc, G. S., Headrick, L. A., Moore, S. M., Barton, A. J., Donalsky, M. A., & Madigosky, W. S. (2012). *Fundamentals of health care improvement* (2nd ed.). Oakbrook Terrace, IL.: Joint Commission Resources and Institute for Healthcare Improvement.

OPM.gov. (n.d.) Performance management: Teams. Retrieved from https://www.opm.gov/policy-data-oversight/performance-management/teams

Pearson, A., Porritt, K., Doran, D., Vincent, L., Craig, D., Tucker, D., & Long, L. (2006). A systematic review of evidence on the professional practice of the nurse and developing and sustaining a healthy work environment in health care. *International Journal of Evidence Based Healthcare, 4*(3), 221–261.

Rastkar, R., Zweig, S., Delzell, J. E., & Davis, K. (2002). Nurse care coordination of ambulatory frail elderly in an academic setting. *Case Manager, 13*(1), 59–61.

Rogers, S. (2008). Inpatient care coordination for patients with diabetes. *Diabetes Spectrum, 21*(4), 273–275.

Schmalenberg, C., & Kramer, M. (2008). Essentials of a productive nurse work environment. *Nursing Research, 57*(1), 2–13.

Skillings, L. N., & MacLeod, D. (2009). The patient care coordinator role: An innovative delivery model for transforming acute care and improving patient outcomes. *Nursing Administration Quarterly, 33*(4), 296–300.

TeamSTEPPS. (n.d.). TeamSTEPPS®: National implementation. Retrieved from http://teamstepps.ahrq.gov/

Vanriel, M. K., Bellack, J. P., & O'Neil, E. (2012). Nurses in the C-Suite: Leadership beyond chief nurse. *Nursing Administration Quarterly, 36*(1), 5–11.

Wong, C. A, & Cummings, G. G. (2007). The relationship between nursing leadership and patient outcomes: A systematic review. *Journal of Nursing Management, 15*, 508–521.

Section 3

Improving Quality Through Effective Care Coordination

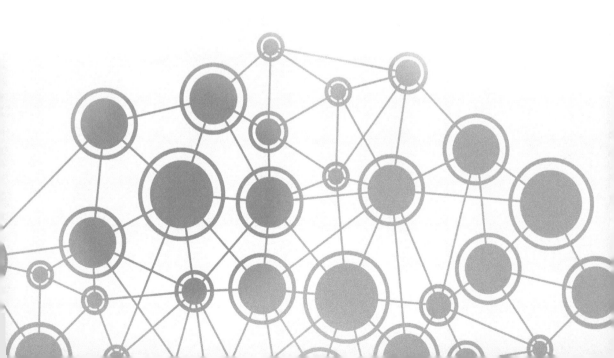

Chapter 7

Care Coordination and Reducing Avoidable Hospital Stays

Karen Jiggins Colorafi, MBA, RN, CPEHR, CPHIT;
Nan M. Solomons, MS; and Gerri Lamb, PhD, RN, FAAN

Changing the way we think about and use our hospitals is a central component of the national quality agenda in the United States. In spite of years of effort to shift attention and resources from acute care to primary prevention and health promotion, hospitals have continued to consume most of our healthcare resources. Today, there is a concerted national effort to align healthcare policy, clinical practice, and innovative use of technology to reduce unnecessary hospital admissions and readmissions. Care coordination is vital to this work. In this chapter, we explore the range of hospital- and community-based care coordination programs that are being used to reduce avoidable hospitalizations and the role that nurses play within these programs.

BACKGROUND AND SIGNIFICANCE

The national quality spotlight has focused on the overuse of hospital services and particularly on preventable hospital readmissions. A preventable hospital readmission is defined as an admission related to a previous admission which could have been avoided (Goldfield et al., 2008). Ambulatory care sensitive conditions such as pneumonia, chronic obstructive pulmonary disease, congestive heart failure, asthma, and diabetes are examples of conditions which research shows can be treated more safely and effectively in the primary care setting at a lower cost (Zeng et al., 2006).

Preventing hospital readmissions is a complex issue in which patient, provider, and access to care may contribute to the need for hospitalization (Boutwell, Griffen, Hwu, & Shannon, 2009). Current estimates of preventable readmissions range from a low of 5% to a high of 79% of initial hospital admissions, depending on how preventable readmission was defined and measured. In general, readmissions rates have hovered around

19% in the U.S. (van Walraven, Bennett, Jennings, Austin, & Forster, 2011). This suggests that about 2 in 10 patients admitted to a U.S. hospital could have been safely managed in the community. Admitting or readmitting patients who do not need to be hospitalized increases the risk of exposure to adverse outcomes including infections, falls, and medication errors (Office of the Inspector General, 2010; Golden, Tewary, Dang, & Roos, 2010).

Unnecessary hospitalizations are extremely expensive. Patients admitted with ambulatory sensitive conditions accounted for 4.4 million hospitalizations, $29 billion in total costs, and 10% of total hospital expenditures for the period between 1999 and 2004 (Boutwell et al., 2009). Medicare spending for inpatients as a result of readmission was $17.5 billion in 2010 (Brennan, 2012). Given these figures, it is not surprising that the Centers for Medicare and Medicaid Services (CMS) instituted penalties for 30-day readmissions in 2013 for three of the most common ambulatory sensitive conditions: heart attack, heart failure, and pneumonia.

Spurred by recognition of the serious nature and cost implications of unnecessary readmissions, and the introduction of payment incentives, hospitals and their community partners are actively seeking new processes and programs to reduce readmissions. The national focus on reducing hospitalizations, more than any other outcome, has vaulted care coordination into the national quality spotlight. Well-known care coordination programs are being rediscovered and refined; new programs, often based on combinations of care coordination interventions developed over many years, have emerged. In the following section, we describe these programs and their impact on reducing hospital readmissions.

REVIEW OF THE LITERATURE

The following program descriptions have been categorized into hospital-initiated and community-initiated programs. Program descriptions are organized to orient the reader to the roles and responsibilities of the care coordinator, key interventions, and significant outcomes. Care coordination programs published in peer-reviewed journals within the last ten years (2002–2012) were reviewed and included when they were nurse-led and measured readmission or the cost associated with hospital utilization as outcomes. Environmental scans were performed to locate non-academic interventions. Interventions conducted in countries other than the United States were excluded.

Hospital-Initiated Programs

In this section, we review programs with care coordination interventions that are initiated within the hospital to reduce subsequent hospital readmissions. Many of these programs continue into post-acute and long-term care settings for a defined period of time, such as 30 or 60 days. The most common care coordination interventions within these hospital-initiated programs are early identification of risk for readmission, patient education, medication reconciliation, and timely discharge communication to the next point of care (Hess et al., 2010; B. Jack et al., 2008; Koehler et al., 2009; Parry, Min, Chugh, Chalmers, & Coleman, 2009).

- *Transitional Care for the Elderly* (Naylor et al., 2004): The goal of the Transitional Care Model is to improve health outcomes and reduce hospital readmissions for individuals with multiple chronic conditions (MCC), including congestive heart failure. In this model, an advanced practice nurse (APRN) initiates discharge planning during the hospital stay for randomized intervention patients. The APRN visits with the patient and family in their homes within 24 hours of discharge and weekly for the first month post-discharge. There are a minimum of eight home visits per patient during the 12 weeks of the trial, during which APRNs pay special attention to symptom management. The results of numerous studies testing this model have found reductions in readmission rates (104 vs. 162 at 52 weeks, p=.047) with an overall decline in hospital costs ($7,636 vs. $12,481, p=.02) and improved quality of life (at 12 weeks, p<.05) for patients in the intervention group compared to the control group.

- *Chronically Ill Patients in ICU* (Daly, Douglas, Genet Kelley, O'Toole, & Montenegro, 2005; Douglas, Daly, Genet Kelley, O'Toole, & Montenegro, 2007): This program focuses on reducing hospitalizations for intensive care patients by adding a disease management program to the usual discharge process. An APRN functioning as the case manager conducts all discharge planning activities, including leading team meetings in the hospital prior to discharge. The APRN meets with the patient and family within 48 hours of discharge in the patient's home and creates a patient-centered clinical summary with a plan of care for all caregivers. The APRN conducts routine visits twice in the first week post-discharge, weekly for the next three weeks, and at least bi-weekly for the remainder of the two month study period, for a minimum total of eight home visits. Compared with the randomized control group, patients receiving the intervention had improved physical health-related quality-of-life scores (p=.02). While there was not a significant difference in readmission rates between the intervention and control groups, the intervention group had significantly shorter lengths of stay during subsequent readmissions (mean of 5.77 fewer days) and a reduction in costs (average savings of $19,705 per patient).

- *Discharge Education and Utilization in Heart Failure* (Koelling, Johnson, Cody, & Aaronson, 2005): This program focuses on reducing hospital readmissions for individuals hospitalized with heart failure (HF). All patients receive standardized written discharge instructions from staff nurses including information about medication, diet, daily weight, activity, and follow-up appointments. Patients randomized to the intervention group also receive an hour long, one-on-one teaching session with a nurse educator who illustrates the physiology of heart failure and how diuretics work. Specific instructions about sodium and fluid restriction are provided along with a copy of HF treatment guidelines written in laymen's terms. An emphasis is placed on the rationale for self-care behaviors. Patients receiving the intervention had fewer deaths and hospitalizations (50 vs. 74 patients, p=.018), a shorter length of stay during subsequent hospitalizations (34 vs. 54 days, p=.014), and had a lower risk of rehospitalization for HF (16 vs. 33 patients, p=.015) during the 180-day follow up period. Intervention patients had a lower cost of care by $2,823 per patient (p=.035).

- *Better Outcomes for Older Adults through Safe Transitions (Project BOOST)* (Society of Hospital Medicine, 2008): The goal of Project BOOST is to redesign hospital workflow using evidence-based processes to reduce readmissions. Using quality improvement processes, workflow and clinician communications are standardized using templates and checklists. Patients are assessed for readmission risk throughout their hospital stay using the General Assessment of Preparedness (GAP) tool. Implementing BOOST is a yearlong mentored process requiring buy-in at all levels of the organization. Preliminary outcomes available on the BOOST website show reductions between 50 and 60% in readmission rates; however, to date there are no published outcomes in the peer-reviewed literature (Society of Hospital Medicine, 2008).

- *State Action on Avoidable Rehospitalization* (STAAR) (Boutwell et al., 2011): The goal of this program is to integrate clinical and policy interventions to reduce rehospitalizations. In this program, service organizations across the full continuum of care work together with state agencies to reduce barriers to successful hospital discharges. Within the hospital, interventions include engaging patients and family, discharge planning, medication reconciliation, and communication with community-based providers. State agencies are engaged in building incentives to improve access to community-based services needed for self-care after hospitalization. Although no outcomes have been reported to date, the planned measures include readmission rates, timeliness of post-discharge communication and appointment-making, patient and family satisfaction with transitional care, and use of community-based services.

■ *Project Re-Engineered Discharge (Project RED)* (Jack et al., 2009): This program seeks to re-engineer the existing discharge process. Standardized procedures are followed for patient education regarding medications, tests, follow-up visits, and the timely transfer of documentation. At discharge, staff nurses enter information about discharge plans into a software program that produces a customized discharge education booklet for each patient. Patients review the booklet while interacting with a conversational agent (or nurse avatar) on a computer screen while in bed. The conversational agent, named Louise, teaches patients about their new medications, self-management strategies, and plans for follow-up. Throughout the session, patients answer questions embedded within the program which demonstrate how well they comprehend the material. Patients can take as much time as they want with the material. Patients randomized to the intervention group had a lower rate of hospital utilization than those receiving usual care (0.314 vs. 0.451 visits per person per month, p=.0009) in the 30-day period post-discharge. Patients were satisfied with the discharge avatar, stating that Louise never talked down to them and explained more than other healthcare professionals who appeared to always be in a hurry.

In summary, a number of different types of programs using care coordination interventions have been initiated in hospitals to reduce readmissions. Some, but not all, of these programs have had the desired impact along with improvements in patient satisfaction and quality of life. Most focus on patient education about medications and chronic illness management while enhancing transfer of information to post-acute providers. Comparisons among programs are difficult to make due to differences in target populations, study design, and outcome measures (Naylor, Aiken, Kurtzman, Olds, & Hirschman, 2011; Rennke et al., 2013; van Walraven et al., 2011). Initial results are promising but more research is needed to achieve consistent outcomes with a broader range of patient populations. Most intervention programs target a specific condition, which is representative of just 10% of hospitalized patients. There is no evidence of program efficacy for the 90% of patients who manage multiple chronic conditions at discharge (Burke & Coleman, 2013; Greenwald & Jack, 2007; Laugaland et al., 2012; Mittler et al., 2013; Nosbusch, Weiss, & Bobay, 2011; Rennke et al., 2013).

Community-Initiated Programs

The programs included in this section are initiated in the community setting and have a goal of keeping patients as healthy as possible in various independent settings in order to avoid unnecessary admission and readmission. The most common care coordination interventions within community settings include a great deal of patient education regarding medication and self-management strategies, as well as nurse-facilitated communication among members of the patient's healthcare team. The community-initiated programs are presented in a similar format to hospital-initiated programs whereby individual program descriptions are organized to orient the reader to the design of the program, primary outcome measures, and results of the program.

- *Exercise in Senior Center* (Leveille et al., 1998): The goal of this program is to reduce risk factors for further disability with physical activity, promote social activation, and enhance medical management of community-based older adults in cooperation with their primary care provider. Over the course of one year in an average of three sessions, a part time geriatric-trained APRN meets with randomized intervention patients and develops a health management plan, teaches self-management strategies, and encourages patients to participate in a wide range of physical activities (swimming, dancing, strength training, tai chi, etc.) available at the senior center. Patients attend the seven-week Chronic Disease Self -Management course. Control group patients are given a tour of the senior center and presented with the opportunity to participate in any of the activities that intervention patients were offered. The intervention group had lower rehospitalization rates over the course of a year (38% year vs. 69%, p=.083), shorter lengths of stay when hospitalized (33 vs. 116, p=.049), fewer disability days, reduced use of psychoactive medications, and higher levels of physical activity.

- *Care Transitions* (Coleman, Parry, Chalmers, & Min, 2006; Coleman et al., 2004): The goal of this program was to encourage older adults and their caregivers to have a more active role during care transitions (leaving the hospital for the community), thereby reducing readmissions. In this program, a registered nurse, sometimes an APRN, referred to as a care transition coach, helps the patient with medication management, instructs on the use of a personalized health record, educates on signs and symptoms of worsening disease, and encourages appropriate primary care and specialist follow-up. The quasi-experimental study (matching intervention patients to administrative controls) found lower rates of readmission in intervention patients at 30 days, 90 days (aOR: 0.43, 95%, 0.25–0.72), and 180 days (aOR: 0.57, 95%, 0.36–0.92). A second randomized controlled trial found lower readmission rates at 30 days (8.3 vs. 11.9, p=.048), as well as 90 days (16.7 vs. 22.5, p=.04), and a reduction in mean hospital costs ($2,058 vs. $2,546, p=.049) for intervention patients over control patients.

- *Nurse Care Management* (Dorr et al., 2006; Dorr et al, 2008): This program was designed to carefully address the six elements of the chronic care model, thereby sustaining health in the community and avoiding rehospitalization. Nurse care managers (as opposed to *case* managers) use a specially designed patient worksheet within an electronic care management tracking system. Nurse care managers make personal visits and telephone calls with patients, communicate with specialists, conduct team meetings, provide assistance with medications, and conduct general coordination activities. Intervention patients, matched with administrative controls receiving usual care in the quasi-experimental design, had lower mortality (6.2% vs. 10.6%, p<.05) and rehospitalization (21% vs. 24%, p<.050) rates one year following the intervention.

- *Case Management by Locus of Control* (Krause et al., 2006): This program was designed to educate and empower patients with chronic illnesses based on the Locus of Control theory. Each patient is assigned a primary registered nurse advocate who works with a single primary physician and behavioral counselor to create a care plan for the patient. The nurse engages in regular meetings with the team, as well as the patient and family. The nurse coordinates the care for the patient, performs compliance tracking, and conducts group education sessions. In this pre-and post-test design, intervention patients reported improvements in physical functioning (p=.02), the amount of time spent exercising (p<.001), perception of well-being (p<.001), self-efficacy (p=.04), and satisfaction (p<.001) but not in locus of control (p=.061) after one year of program participation.

Readmissions were not specifically measured in this study but healthcare costs were. Estimated costs were compared with actual costs to yield a mean difference of $25,209.75 (p<.01).

■ *After Discharge Care Management of Low Income Frail Elderly* **(AD-Life)** (Wright, 2007): In this program, low-income, at-risk elderly patients are identified upon admission by an APRN who facilitates discharge planning throughout the hospitalization. The APRN leads a multidisciplinary team that includes the patient, RN care manager, pharmacist, social worker, and geriatrician. They evaluate evidence-based protocols, develop a care plan, and communicate with the primary care provider (PCP) to provide ongoing follow up. RN care managers visit the PCP at least once for 15 minutes to discuss the care plan for each patient. The PCP is reimbursed for this visit. Results from the feasibility study comparing the year prior to admission and the year post-admission for each patient reported decreased hospital readmissions per 1,000 patients and lower cost of care of $1,000 less per patient per month. The project team recently completed a three year randomized controlled trial and findings have not yet been published (Colorafi & Wright, personal communication).

■ *Aging in Place* (Marek, Adams, Stetzer, Popejoy, & Rantz, 2010; Marek et al., 2005; Marek, Stetzer, Adams, Popejoy, & Rantz, 2012; Marek, Popejoy, Petroski, & Rantz, 2006): This program was developed at the University of Missouri to test an alternative delivery model of community-based, long-term care for Medicare and Medicaid patients and is discussed in more detail in Chapter 12. In this program, older adults receive care coordination services from a geriatrics-prepared registered nurse under the supervision of an APRN. All recipients have an individualized home assessment and a personalized plan of care that is reviewed with patients and families no less than once per month during a home visit. Additional RN activities include medication management and coordination of other services as needed such as physical therapy, homemaking, or personal care. Home visits range from weekly to monthly depending on patient needs.

In a retrospective cohort design that compared patients receiving the intervention to those in another county who did not, the intervention patients had better clinical outcomes in pain, dyspnea, and ADLs (p<.05) at 12 months. Although hospital admission and readmission rates were not measured for this intervention, total per month Medicare costs were lower ($686, p=.04) and Medicaid costs were higher ($203, p=.03) in the intervention group in the 12 months following the intervention. In a subsequent study that compared intervention patients with matched controls in a nursing home group, the total Medicare and Medicaid costs were lower per month ($1,591.61, p<.01) and clinical outcomes in cognition (p=.00 at 6, 12, and 18 months), depression (p=.00 at 6 and 12 months), ADLs (p=.02 at 6 months, p=.04 at 12 months, and p=.00 at 24 months), and incontinence (p=.02 at 24 months) were significantly better in the intervention group.

- *Early Case Management for Older Adults* (Shapiro & Taylor, 2002): The goal of this program was to provide nurse care coordination for low-income, at-risk, community-dwelling elders earlier than it normally would be offered. A registered nurse performs a geriatric assessment during a home visit and creates an initial care plan in cooperation with the patient and family. The case manager meets with the patient at least once every three months, arranging for a wide variety of services including meal delivery, homemaking tasks, chores, personal care, transportation, and respite care. Patients randomized to the intervention group were 82% less likely (OR: .18, p=.029) to be rehospitalized or institutionalized than control patients over the 18-month study.

- *Nurse Care Management for Heart Failure* (DeBusk et al., 2004): This program sought to determine if a nurse-led care coordination program delivered over the telephone would reduce hospitalizations. In addition to usual care, randomized intervention patients receive an in-person initial assessment in a physician's office from a registered nurse who also reviews video-taped and paper-based patient education material. Nurses conduct baseline telephone counseling and initiate subsequent follow-up calls with patients and physicians as needed. At a minimum, nurses schedule calls weekly for six weeks, biweekly for eight weeks, monthly for three months, and bimonthly for another six months. The effect of the intervention at the end of year one was minor. Rates of all-cause hospitalizations and first rehospitalization for heart failure were similar in both groups and not statistically significant.

■ *Standardized Telephone Nurse Case Management* (Riegel et al., 2002): This program also evaluated the effectiveness of telephone-based nurse care coordination in reducing hospitalizations. In this program for recently discharged heart failure patients, a registered nurse provides case management over the telephone. Nurses use a commercially available decision support program to target specific issues known to affect rehospitalization, including medication management, dietary restrictions, and the signs and symptoms of worsening heart failure. Nurses call patients within five days of discharge and schedule subsequent calls at a frequency guided by the software and professional judgment. On average, patients receive 17 calls over a 6 month period, for a minimum of 16 hours of nurse time. At six months, the randomized intervention patients had lower rates of heart failure hospitalization (47.8%, p=.01), fewer inpatient days (46% difference, p=.03), and lower total inpatient costs ($1,192 vs. $2,186 or 45.5%, p=.04) compared with the control group.

■ *Guided Care* (Boult et al., 2011; Boult et al., 2008; Boyd, et al., 2009; Wolff et al., 2010): The goal of this program for patients with chronic disease was to transfer the utilization patterns away from expensive inpatient care to less costly ambulatory services. A registered nurse working out of a physician's office performs a comprehensive initial assessment that includes several standardized measures (nutrition, psychosocial, environmental) and sets individualized goals with the patient and family. Nurses conduct home visits or call patients at least once a month. Motivational interviewing is used to help patients maintain and enforce adherence to their goals which were set during the initial assessment. The Guided Care intervention was found to improve physician–patient interaction (p<.05) and reduce utilization and costs (p<.05) in the pilot project. Despite promising pilot results, the intervention failed to reduce hospital readmissions. The only significant finding was a reduction in episodes of home care (0.70, CI: 95%, 0.31–0.89) and skilled nursing facility admissions (0.53, CI: 95%, 0.31–0.89) among randomized intervention patients. An 18-month follow up reported that intervention patients self-rated the quality of their chronic care more highly than control patients (2.13, CI: 95%, 1.30–3.50) and that family caregivers reported a higher quality of their recipients' chronic illness care (0.40, CI: 95%, 0.14–0.67) when their family member was a part of the intervention group.

■ *GRACE* (Counsell et al., 2007; Counsell, Callahan, Tu, Stump, & Arling, 2009): This program tested the effectiveness of a geriatric care management model for low-income older adults. APRNs and social workers provide in-home assessment and case management for common geriatric conditions over a period of two years using standard protocols developed by physicians involved in the GRACE (Geriatric Resources for Assessment and Care of Elders) program, which is effective in improving quality of care and outcomes. The care plan developed by the APRN is reviewed with an interdisciplinary team and implemented through in-home visits and telephone calls. Each patient receives a minimum of one initial home visit and one telephone follow-up call each month. Patients randomized to the intervention group had improvements in clinical outcomes at 24 months compared with control group patients, including general health (p=.045), vitality (p<.001), social functioning (p=.008), and mental health (p=.001). Cumulative rates of emergency room visits at 24 months were lower for intervention patients than controls (1,445 vs. 1,748, p=.03), but the rate of hospital readmissions was not significantly different between groups (700 vs. 740, p=.66). Further analysis dividing all patients into low- and high-risk groups demonstrated a reduction in hospital admissions for the high-risk intervention patients (396 vs. 705, p=.03) at 24 months when compared with high-risk controls.

In summary, a wide variety of program approaches have been utilized in the community in order to reduce rates of hospital readmissions. Not all programs were successful in decreasing hospital utilization among intervention groups. Community-initiated programs are more likely to be run by a registered nurse versus an APRN, are designed to keep people as healthy as possible in their own setting, and encourage the use of less expensive outpatient resources for ongoing management. Patient education and frequent follow up are core elements of community-initiated programs. The programs measure a wide variety of clinical, utilization, and cost outcomes using a variety of standardized measures and techniques, making comparison between studies difficult. More research is needed to identify the mechanism that makes one community-initiated program more impactful than another.

IMPLICATIONS OF NURSE-LED CARE COORDINATION PROGRAMS

In this section, we review various aspects of the nurse-led care coordination programs previously described that influence preventable readmissions. Some of these programs have consistent impact on reducing readmissions and others do not. The reviews we have conducted indicate that nurses play pivotal roles in care coordination efforts and can have a significant impact on reducing preventable readmission rates.

Patient Education

Every care coordination program reviewed in this chapter included patient education. Nurses taught patients and their families about their diseases, how to recognize symptoms, when and where to go for appropriate help, and built a plan of care that was congruent with patient, family, and provider goals. In a recent review of Medicare demonstration projects (community-initiated), nurses in care coordination interventions that significantly reduced readmissions were found to utilize behavior change and motivational interviewing techniques to adapt evidenced-based education to the patient's preferences and stage of illness (Brown et al., 2012). Increasing patient knowledge about one's illnesses and the ability to manage chronic disease was a foundational element of most programs.

Self-Management of Patients and Families

Through education and coaching, nurses promoted patient and family self-management strategies. Nurses helped patients to develop skills and self-regulation capacities that enhanced their ability to manage their conditions appropriately. A substantial amount of time was spent on medication management in particular. Older adults receiving care coordination services often have a significant burden of chronic disease that is managed with a myriad of medications. Nurses in successful programs manage medication lists from several reliable sources and have ready access to APRNs, physicians, and pharmacists when discrepancies arose. Nurses in the programs we reviewed spend a great deal of time discerning what should be on the current medication list among past, current, and newly prescribed medications; communicating with pharmacists to ensure patient access to appropriate medications; and teaching the patient why and how to take the medication. Medication management is a time-consuming and vital part of the programs we reviewed.

Communication within Care Teams

Successful care coordination programs created opportunities for nurses and providers to work together regularly within and across care environments. Sometimes programs were designed so that a specific nurse could work with a specific provider or unit so that all patients in one panel were covered by the same two people. This greatly increased the opportunities for interaction among clinicians, which eventually increased the trust they had in each other. Real-time communication between clinicians has been found to decrease readmissions and provides an opportunity to share patient details that are not part of the written summary (Hess et al., 2010). This is especially relevant when patients transition from the hospital to a community setting. Frequent meetings with professional caregivers across the continuum provide opportunities to work out logistical and process issues that can contribute to hospital readmissions (Cortes, Robinson, & Street, 2004). One of the nurses' most important roles in these programs was to serve as a communications hub, ensuring that all of the patient's providers have key information about the patient (ANA, 2012; Brown et al., 2012; Quality and Safety Education for Nurses, 2012). Nurses in these programs spent a significant amount of time on the phone, writing emails, sending faxes, and updating shared patient records; they were masterful communicators.

Amount of Nurse–Patient Interaction

One of the most highly variable factors across programs was the amount of time nurses and patients spent together. Many of the programs we have reviewed in this chapter incorporate regular home visits and/or telephone calls to routinely check in with patients. The intensity or dose of the care coordination intervention required to reduce preventable readmissions deserves further consideration. Regular visits in the patient's home, more than visits in a physician's office or visits over the telephone, may be an important factor in avoiding rehospitalization. Community-initiated programs have more opportunity for consistent face time with patients. Hospital-initiated programs adhere to this principle by providing extra time with an educator, conversational agent, pharmacist, or APRN prior to discharge.

Innovation and Study Design

Although research into care coordination has been ongoing for many decades, there is considerable opportunity for innovation. Several programs that achieved significant results contain unique elements, such as the conversational agent or avatar, an exercise component, the addition of a social worker to the care coordination team, and the provision of homemaking or personal services. Overall, care coordination programs appear to have a significant impact on the lives of patients, who are regularly more satisfied with their health care, enjoy better quality of life, and improved physical and mental functioning.

Measurement of Care Coordination Outcomes

Perhaps the most problematic element of this review was evaluating and interpreting the multiple instruments used to measure various outcomes. Much like the Chronic Disease Self-Management Program uses a set of standardized instruments to evaluate its effectiveness across populations, settings, disease states, and even cultures (Lorig et al., 2010), care coordination programs need to incorporate standardized performance measures, including measures of patient and family experience and satisfaction. The National Institute for Nursing Research, with input from the National Institutes of Health, has created a strategic plan which calls for the widespread use of the national bank of Patient Outcome Measurement Information System (PROMIS) instruments. The use of these valid and reliable standardized tools will allow researchers to measure a variety of health outcomes across multiple diseases (NINR, 2006). Tools such as these will streamline future comparisons and allow for more sophisticated analysis of the variables that contribute to outcomes.

Finally, structures and incentives within our current healthcare system impact the effectiveness of care coordination across the continuum of care and, in turn, are impacting hospital readmission rates. Care coordination interventions may be delivered in settings that have incentives that run counter to the goal of reducing preventable hospitalizations. Emerging delivery models, such as Patient Centered Healthcare, Medical Homes, or Accountable Care organizations offer the promise for new systems that fully incorporate and optimize care coordination interventions.

CONCLUSION

Studies of care coordination models conducted over many years demonstrate the contribution of nurse care coordination to reducing preventable hospitalizations and their associated costs to patients, families, and the healthcare system. Importantly, these studies serve as a rich repository of nursing knowledge about nurse care coordination interventions that are central to effectiveness, including key roles in communication, education, and establishing on-going relationships in which nurses "know" their patients and their needs and preferences (Bowles, Faust, & Naylor, 2003). Current initiatives to standardize measurement of care coordination structures, processes, and outcomes are an important step in advancing the practice and impact of nurse care coordination.

REFERENCES

American Nurses Association (ANA). (2012). *The value of nursing care coordination: A white paper of the American Nurses Association*. Retrieved from http://www.nursingworld.org/carecoordinationwhitepaper

Boult, C., Reider, L., Frey, K., Leff, B., Boyd, C. M., Wolff, J. L., ... Scharfstein, D. (2008). Early effects of "guided care" on the quality of health care for multimorbid older persons: A cluster-randomized controlled trial. *Journals of Gerontology Series A: Biological Sciences and Medical Sciences, 63*(3), 321–327.

Boult, C., Redier, L., Leff, B., Frick, K., Boyd, C., Wolff, J., ... Scharfstein, S. (2011). The effect of guided care teams on the use of health services. *Archives of Internal Medicine, 171*(5), 460–466.

Boutwell, A., Griffen, F., Hwu, S., & Shannon, D. (2009). Effective interventions to reduce rehospitalizations: A compendium of 15 promising interventions. In *Institute for Healthcare Improvement* (Ed.). Cambridge: Institute for Healthcare Improvement.

Boutwell, A., Johnson, M. B., Rutherford, P., Watson, S. R., Vecchioni, N., Auerbach, B. S., ... Wagner, C. (2011). An early look at a four-state initiative to reduce avoidable hospital readmissions. *Health Aff (Millwood), 30*(7), 1272–1280. doi: 10.1377/hlthaff.2011.0111

Boyd, C., Reider, L., Frey, K., Scharstein, D., Leff, B., Wolff, J., ... Boult, C. (2009). The effects of guided care on the perceived quality of health care for multi-morbid older persons: 18-month outcomes from a cluster-randomized controlled trial. *Journal of General Internal Medicine, 25*(3), 235–242. doi: 10.1007/s11606-009-1192-5

Brennan, N. (2012). National medicare readmission findings: Recent data and trends. In *Office of Information Products and Data Analytics Centers for Medicare and Medicare Services* (Ed.): Baltimore, MD: Centers for Medicare and Medicaid Services.

Brown, R., Peikes, D., Peterson, G., Schore, J., & Razafindrakoto, C. (2012). Six features of Medicare coordinated care demonstration programs that cut hospital admission of high-risk patients. *Health Affairs, 31*(6), 1156–1166. doi: 10.1377/hlthaff.2012.0393

Burke, R. E., & Coleman, E. A. (2013). Interventions to decrease hospital readmissions: Keys for cost-effectiveness. *Journal of the American Medical Association: Internal Medicine, 173*(8), 695–698. doi: 10.1001/jamainternmed.2013.171

Coleman, E. A., Parry, C., Chalmers, S., & Min, S. (2006). The care transitions intervention: Results of a randomized controlled trial. *Archives of Internal Medicine, 166*, 1822–1828.

Coleman, E. A., Smith, J. D., Frank, J. C., Min, S., Parry, C., & Kramer, A. M. (2004). Preparing patients and caregivers to participate in care delivered across settings: The care transitions intervention. *Journal of the American Geriatrics Society, 52*(11), 1817–1825. doi: 10.1111/j.1532-5415.2004.52504.x

Cortes, T. A., Wexler, S., & Fitzpatrick, J. J. (2004). The transition of elderly patients between hospitals and nursing homes. *Journal of Gerontological Nursing*, 10–15.

Counsell, S. R., Callahan, C. M., Clark, D. O., Tu, W., Buttar, A. B., Stump, T. E., & Ricketts, G. D. (2007). Geriatric care management for low-income seniors: A randomized controlled trial. *Journal of the American Medical Association, 298*(22), 2623–2633. doi: 10.1001/jama.298.22.2623

Counsell, S., Callahan, C., Tu, W., Stump, T., & Arling, G. (2009). Cost analysis of the geriatric resources for assessment and care of elders care management intervention. *Journal of the American Geriatrics Society, 57*, 1420–1426. doi: 10.1111/j.1532-5415.2009.02383.x

Daly, B., Douglas, S., Genet Kelley, C., O'Toole, E., & Montenegro, H. (2005). Trial of a disease management program to reduce hospital readmissions of the chronically critically ill. *Chest, 128*(2), 507–517.

DeBusk, R. F., Miller, N. H., Parker, K. M., Bandura, A., Kraemer, H. C., Cher, D. J., … Greenwald, G. (2004). Care management for low-risk patients with heart failure: A randomized, controlled trial. *Annals of Internal Medicine, 141*(8), 606–613.

Dorr, D., Wilcox, A., Brunker, C., Burdon, R., & Donnelly, S. (2008). The effect of technology-supported, multidisease care management on the mortality and hospitalization of seniors. *Journal of the American Geriatrics Society, 56*, 2195–2202. doi: 10.1111/j.1532-5415.2008.02005.x

Dorr, D., Wilcox, A., Burns, L., Brukner, C., Narus, S., & Clayton, P. (2006). Implementing a multidisease chronic care model in primary care using people and technology. *Disease Management, 9*(1), 1–15.

Douglas, S., Daly, B., Genet Kelley, C., O'Toole, E., & Montenegro, H. (2007). Chronically critically ill patients: Health related quality of life and resource use after a disease management intervention. *American Journal of Critical Care, 16*(5), 447–457.

Golden, A. G., Tewary, S., Dang, S., & Roos, B. A. (2010). Care management's challenges and opportunities to reduce the rapid rehospitalization of frail community-dwelling older adults. *Gerontologist, 50*(4), 451–458. doi: 10.1093/geront/gnq015

Goldfield, N. I., McCullough, E. C., Hughes, J. S., Tang, A. M., Eastman, B., Rawlins, L. K., & Averill, R. F. (2008). Identifying potentially preventable readmissions. *Health Care Financing Review, 30*(1), 75–91.

Greenwald, J., & Jack, B. (2007). Preventing the preventable: Reducing hospitalizations through coordinated, patient-centered discharge processes. *Professional Case Management, 14*(3), 135–140.

Hess, D. R., Tokarczyk, A., O'Malley, M., Gavaghan, S., Sullivan, J., & Schmidt, U. (2010). The value of adding a verbal report to written handoffs on early readmission following prolonged respiratory failure. *Chest, 138*(6), 1475–1479.

Jack, B., Greenwald, J., Forsythe, S., O'Donnell, J., Johnson, A., Schipelliti, L., … Chetty, V. K. (2008). *Developing the tools to administer a comprehensive hospital discharge program: The ReEngineered Discharge (RED) Program advances in patient safety: New directions and alternative approaches (Vol. 3: Performance and tools)*. Rockville MD: Agency for Healthcare Research and Quality.

Jack, B. W., Chetty, V. K., Anthony, D., Greenwald, J. L., Sanchez, G. M., Johnson, A. E., … Culpepper, L. (2009). A reengineered hospital discharge program to decrease rehospitalization. *Annals of Internal Medicine, 150*(3), 178–187.

Koehler, B. E., Richter, K. M., Youngblood, L., Cohen, B. A., Prengler, I. D., Cheng, D., & Masica, A. L. (2009). Reduction of 30-day postdischarge hospital readmission or emergency department (ED) visit rates in high-risk elderly medical patients through delivery of a targeted care bundle. *Journal of Hospital Medicine, 4*, 211–218. doi: 10.1002/jhm.427

Koelling, T. M., Johnson, M. L., Cody, R. J., & Aaronson, K. D. (2005). Discharge education improves clinical outcomes in patients with chronic heart failure. *Circulation, 111*, 179–185.

Krause, C., Joyce, S., Curtin, K., Krause, C., Jones, C., Kuhn, M., … Boan, B. (2006). The impact of a multidisciplinary, integrated approach on improving the health and quality of care for individuals dealing with multiple chronic conditions. *American Journal of Orthopsychiatry, 76*(1), 109–114. doi: 10.1037/0002-9432.76.1.109

Laugaland, K., Aase, K., & Barach, P. (2012). Interventions to improve patient safety in transitional care: A review of the evidence. *Work, 41 Suppl 1*, 2915–2924. doi: 10.3233/WOR-2012-0544-2915

Leveille, S., Wagner, E., Davis, C., Grothaus, L., Wallace, J., LoGerfo, M., & Kent, D. (1998). Preventing disability and managing chronic illness in frail older adults: A randomized trial of a community-based partnership with primary care. *Journal of the American Geriatrics Society, 46*, 1191–1198.

Lorig, K., Ritter, P., Laurent, D., Plant, K., Green, M., Blue Bird, V., & Case, S. (2010). Online diabetes self-management program. *Diabetes Care, 33*(6), 1275–1281.

Marek, K., Adams, S., Stetzer, F., Popejoy, L., & Rantz, M. (2010). The relationship of community-based nurse care coordination to costs in the Medicare and Medicaid programs. *Research in Nursing and Health, 33*, 235–242. doi: 10.1002/nur.20378

Marek, K., Popejoy, L., Petroski, G., Mehr, D., Rantz, M., & Lin, W. C. (2005). Clinical outcome of aging in place. *Nursing Research, 54*(3), 202–211.

Marek, K., Stetzer, F., Adams, S., Popejoy, L., & Rantz, M. (2012). Aging in place verus nursing home care: Comparison of costs to medicare and medicaid. *Research in Gerontological Nursing, 5*(2), 123–129.

Marek, K., Popejoy, L., Petroski, G., & Rantz, M. (2006). Nurse care coordination in community-based long-term care. *Journal of Nursing Scholarship, 38*(1), 80–86.

Mittler, J. N., O'Hora, J. L., Harvey, J. B., Press, M. J., Volpp, K. G., & Scanlon, D. P. (2013). Turning readmission reduction policies into results: Some lessons from a multistate initiative to reduce readmissions. *Population Health Manaement, 16*(4): 255–260. doi: 10.1089/pop.2012.0087

NINR. (2006). Focus on NINR and the NIH Roadmap: A focus paper on NINR research directions and advances. Retrieved from http://www.ninr.nih.gov/sites/www.ninr.nih.gov/files/RoadmapFocusFINAL113006.pdf

Naylor, M. D. (2012). Advancing high value transitional care: The central role of nursing and its leadership. *Nursing Administration Quarterly April/June, 36*(2), 115–126.

Naylor, M. D., Aiken, L. H., Kurtzman, E. T., Olds, D. M., & Hirschman, K. B. (2011). The importance of transitional care in achieving health reform. *Health Affairs, 30*(4), 746–754.

Naylor, M. D., Brooten, D. A., Campbell, R. L., Maislin, G., McCauley, K. M., & Schwartz, J. S. (2004). Transitional care of older adults hospitalized with heart failure: A randomized, controlled trial [corrected] [published erratum appears in *Journal of the Ameican Geriatrics Society, 52*(7):1228]. *Journal of the American Geriatrics Society, 52*(5), 675–684.

Nosbusch, J. M., Weiss, M. E., & Bobay, K. L. (2011). An integrated review of the literature on challenges confronting the acute care staff nurse in discharge planning. *Journal of Clinical Nursing, 20*(5–6), 754–774. doi: 10.1111/j.1365-2702.2010.03257.x

Office of the Inspector General. (2010). *Adverse events in hospitals: National incidents among Medicare beneficiaries.* Washington, DC: Department of Health and Human Services.

Parry, C., Min, S. J., Chugh, A., Chalmers, S., & Coleman, E. A. (2009). Further application of the care transitions intervention: Results of a randomized controlled trial conducted in a fee-for-service setting. *Home Health Care Services Qaurtlery, 28*(2–3), 84–99. doi: 10.1080/01621420903155924

Quality and Safety Education for Nurses. (2012). Competency KSAs (Prelicensure). Retrieved from http://www.qsen.org/ksas_prelicensure.php

Rennke, S., Nguyen, O. K., Shoeb, M. H., Magan, Y., Wachter, R. M., & Ranji, S. R. (2013). Hospital-initiated transitional care interventions as a patient safety strategy: A systematic review. *Annals of Internal Medicine, 158*(5 (Part 2)), 433–440.

Riegel, B., Carlson, B., Kopp, Z., LePetri, B., Glaser, D., & Unger, A. (2002). Effect of a standardized nurse case-management telephone intervention on resource use in patients with chronic heart failure. *Archives of Internal Medicine, 162*(6), 705–712.

Shapiro, A., & Taylor, M. (2002). Effects of a community-based early intervention program on the subjective well-being, institutionalization, and mortality of low-income elders. *The Gerentologist, 42*(3), 334–341.

Society of Hospital Medicine. (2008). BOOSTing Care Transitions Resource Room. Retrieved from http://www.hospitalmedicine.org/resourceroomredesign/rr_caretransitions/ct_home.cfm

van Walraven, C., Bennett, C., Jennings, A., Austin, P. C., & Forster, A. J. (2011). Proportion of hospital readmissions deemed avoidable: A systematic review. *Canadian Medical Association Journal, 183*(7), E391–E402. doi: 10.1503/cmaj.110448

Wolff, J., Giovannetti, E., Boyd, C., Redier, L., Palmer, S., Scharfstein, D., … Boult, C. (2010). Effects of Guided Care on Family Caregivers. *The Gerentologist, 50*(4), 459–470.

Wright, K. (2007). The AD-Life Trial: Working to integrate medical and psychosocial care management models. *Home Healthcare Nurse, 25*(5), 308–314.

Zeng, F., O'Leary, J. F., Sloss, E. M., Lopez, M. S., Dhanani, N., & Melnick, G. (2006). The effect of medicare health maintenance organizations on hospitalization rates for ambulatory care-sensitive conditions. *Medical Care, 44*(10), 900–907. doi: 10.2307/41219538

Chapter 8

Quality and Safety Outcomes for Patients and Families

Sheila Haas, PhD, RN, FAAN and
Beth Ann Swan, PhD, CRNP, FAAN

Care coordination is at the center of most discussions and seen as a key solution for providing safe, quality care, reducing healthcare costs, improving outcomes by specifically supporting self-care, managing medications, promoting safe practices, and reducing healthcare-acquired conditions, use of emergency departments for care, and readmission to hospitals in less than 30 days post hospital discharge. In the *National Strategy for Quality Improvement in Health Care* report to Congress, "promoting effective communication and coordination of care" is one of six priorities to advance the triple aim of better care, healthy people and communities, and affordable care (AHRQ, 2011).

While there are many definitions of care coordination and transition management, one thing is certain: patients, especially those with complex chronic conditions, need a road map and customized care coordination to navigate our complex care system. As described in earlier chapters, numerous initiatives are underway in the United States to accomplish this. This chapter highlights the relationship between essential care coordination interventions, such as those identified by the Agency for Healthcare Research and Quality (AHRQ) (2012) shown in Table 1, and quality and safety outcomes for patients and families. Selected examples are used to illustrate how care coordination outcomes may be achieved and the implications for nursing practice, education, and research. A logic model is provided to show the connections between registered nurse (RN) competencies for care coordination and transitional care, care coordination interventions and activities performed by the interprofessional care teams, and short-, medium-, and long-term outcomes. The logic model may be used to guide practice, research, and education.

Table 1 Essential Elements of Care Coordination

■ Baseline comprehensive needs assessment
■ Periodically update comprehensive needs assessment
■ Develop an individualized plan of care
■ Routinely update individualized plan of care
■ Facilitate access to medical care and home and community-based services and supports
■ Regularly monitor and communicate

Source: AHRQ, 2012a

CARE COORDINATION INTERVENTIONS AND QUALITY AND SAFETY OUTCOMES

Care coordination is a major strategy for addressing complex health and social issues and improving quality outcomes and performance measures. The body of evidence linking care coordination to important quality outcomes like self-care, medication use, and safety is still small, but growing. Examples of promising areas of research are described below.

Improving Patient Engagement and Self-Care Practices

Individuals, families, and providers' expectations related to self-care and ongoing support must be clear. Care coordination interventions focused on clarifying expectations for self-care and improving competence in self-care activities include:

1. Assessing patients' comprehensive health status—physical, psychological, social, and role function (Aliotta et al., 2008)

2. Developing a plan of care in collaboration with patients and their families (Aliotta et al., 2008)

3. Evaluating their capacity, energy level, and support systems, as well as their readiness, ability, and skills to organize and manage their plan (Swan, 2012)

4. Coaching and educating patients and their families (Aliotta et al., 2008)

5. Empowering patients for self-management (Hibbard & Greene, 2013)

Foundational to the self-care activities required for care coordination is patient activation and engagement. Patient activation "emphasizes patients' willingness and ability to take independent actions to manage their health and care"; whereas patient engagement "denotes a broader concept that includes activation, the interventions designed to increase activation, and patients' resulting behavior" (Hibbard & Greene, 2013, p. 207).

Patient engagement and self-care expectations for patients/families are often compromised by socioeconomic factors, such as: insufficient housing, food, and transportation; low health literacy; and sensory deficits that do not have sufficient remediation such as glasses and hearing aids. Also, patients with no social support, family, or who live alone are often unable to fully provide self-care (Craig, Eby, & Whittington, 2011).

Medication Management

Medication management is a second area requiring a coordinated approach, as well as ongoing management and reconciliation across all settings of care. Care coordination interventions focused on managing medications include:

1. Improving patient's understanding of instructions for newly prescribed, ongoing, or post-discharge medications and understanding of post-discharge instructions including recognizing early warning signs and symptoms

2. Improving access to patient and health information exchange

3. Ongoing communication about any changes in medications; and

4. Using decision aids and reminders (AHRQ, 2012b), as well as establishing a "go-to" resource in their primary setting who can counsel or coach them as medication issues arise before the issues become catastrophic

Some of the medication management patient-centered outcomes to consider include clinical outcomes, quality of life, patient satisfaction, and quality of care. In a recent AHRQ report (2013a), one message was clear: "there is no silver bullet" for improving medication management outcomes and improving medication management does not necessarily mean improvement in other chronic disease outcomes. Recommendations included reducing out-of-pocket medication costs, selecting different interventions based on the patient condition and chronic disease(s), avoiding polypharmacy as much as possible, and establishing medication reconciliation processes/systems. Medication reconciliation systems must include all members of the healthcare team and must address all settings where the patient is receiving care.

Safe Practices

For more than a decade, safe practices have been a focus of healthcare delivery from many perspectives, including patient and families, providers, organizations, researchers, and policymakers. Outcomes associated with safe practices include some very familiar goals, such as reducing rates of infections and reducing falls. Many of the safe practices endorsed by the National Quality Forum (NQF) and the AHRQ, such as medication reconciliation and transitional care, rely on care coordination interventions.

Care coordination interventions focused on safe practices are targeted at reducing patient risk and improving patient safety in inpatient and outpatient settings, including the patients' homes, by involving patients and their families, as well as providers and organizations. From the perspective of patients and families, informed consent and providing information about what to expect before, during, and following a visit, treatment, or procedure is critical so that patients and families are engaged, ready to manage, prepared to coordinate needed care, have the necessary tools and equipment, and are able to recognize and report problems and adverse events. When a patient is returning home, the patient and/or caregiver needs to know what to do and who to call in the case of a problem or adverse event. From the perspective of providers, interprofessional teamwork training and skill building is critical to providing coordinated and safe care across settings.

Healthcare-Acquired Conditions

While reducing healthcare-acquired conditions may seem beyond the realm of care coordination, a focus in the Affordable Care Act (2010) on care coordination and preventive interventions is critical as more patients with central lines, ventilators, and indwelling catheters are cared for in their homes and a variety of outpatient settings. While the focus on reducing healthcare-acquired conditions has been on interventions in hospital settings, it is imperative to move prevention programs beyond inpatient settings. Hand hygiene, influenza prevention, central line-associated bloodstream infection prevention, care of the ventilated patient, multidrug-resistant organism prevention, catheter-associated urinary tract infection prevention, and pressure ulcer prevention are included in the NQF's safe practice set and focus on reducing healthcare-acquired conditions (NQF, 2013).

Care Coordination Models: Targeting Outcomes

Care coordination models have been developed recognizing that coordinating care for individuals with chronic conditions and/or complex healthcare needs now requires new models of care delivery. Care coordination models are intended to achieve the goals described above, prevent the costly consequences of poor management, and improve the short- and long-term quality outcomes for individuals. Ideally, emerging models should include interventions targeted at achieving outcomes associated with effective care coordination.

In the following discussion, we use one popular model of care coordination, the Guided Care Model (Boult, 2008), to illustrate how different care coordination interventions may be associated with quality and safety outcomes. This model was selected to represent a well-tested model and variations in the complexity of patient needs addressed. The Guided Care Model promotes a systematic, planned, team approach toward health and illness with patients at the center of care delivery playing an active role in interactions leading to positive patient outcomes, improved quality of care, and delivery system redesign, as well as use of decision support and clinical information systems. The description of the model includes an overview of expected outcomes and care coordination interventions, as well as an explanation of the hypothesized relationship between the care coordination interventions and quality and safety outcomes.

The Guided Care Model, led by Dr. Chad Boult, is a program that integrates multiple interventions and delivers care through a nurse–physician care partnership to successfully manage chronically ill individuals 65 years and older (Boult, 2008). Targeted outcomes in this model are:

1. An increase in patient physical and mental health, quality of care, and satisfaction with care

2. A decrease in caregiver strain, costs, health, and quality of care

3. An increase in primary care practice satisfaction and organizational dynamics on the part of staff

4. An increase in RN job satisfaction; in addition to reductions in preventable rehospitalization

In this model, most of the care coordination interventions are delivered by a RN based in the primary care setting. The RN visits hospitalized patients within two days of admission to the hospital and two days prior to discharge and then follows the patient into the home to monitor and support self-care practices. Unlike other transitional care models that are time-limited, this primary care-based model offers continuity and an ongoing relationship with chronically-ill adults. Specific Guided Care nurse interventions include:

1. Assessing patient needs and preferences

2. Creating an evidence-based care guide

3. Monitoring the patient proactively

4. Supporting chronic disease self-management

5. Educating and supporting caregivers

6. Communicating with all external care and service providers

7. Facilitating smooth transitions between sites of care

8. Facilitating access to community services (Boyd et al., 2007)

In this model, proactively assessing needs, creating a plan, and supporting monitoring and management are hypothesized as the core factors influencing targeted quality and cost outcomes. Hypothesized relationships among care coordination processes, specific process goals, and outcomes are shown in Table 2 and are described in greater detail in the following section.

Making the Care Coordination and Quality Outcomes Link

Analysis of the interprofessional literature on care coordination and transitional care indicates that many factors need to be considered in establishing a link between care coordination interventions and quality and safety outcomes. These include such elements as the profession or preparation of the individual delivering the interventions, the site or sites of care, and the timeframe for achieving the intended outcomes.

Nurses have played a major role in many of the care coordination models described in the literature. Importantly, several of these models also rely on social workers, physicians, and therapists, as well as family members and community outreach workers. Each group brings a unique set of knowledge and skills to care coordination. The setting for care coordination also may have a significant effect on the type and duration of impact. In recent years, much of the research on care coordination has focused on transitional care to reduce hospitalization and rehospitalization. This work is detailed in the previous chapter. However, there also is a long history of community-based care coordination emphasizing self-care, functional performance, and quality of life in the community (Coburn, Marcantonio, Lazansky, Keller, & Davis, 2012). Each combination of provider, setting, care coordination interventions, and duration may be expected to have shorter- or longer-term effects. Transitional care models, for example, typically are examined for impact at 30 or 60 days. Community-based models, in which care coordinators work with patients and families for prolonged periods, may show effects over months or even years.

With each of these factors and many more at play, it is essential to have models and frameworks to guide how we study the relationship between care coordination and important quality and safety outcomes for patients and families. We developed a specific type of model, called a logic model, that links nurse competencies, care coordination processes, and outcomes (Haas & Swan, 2013). Our model focuses on establishing relationships among these three elements in ambulatory and community settings since these settings offer significant opportunities for nurses to demonstrate their contributions to quality and safety outcomes. In addition to guiding care coordination research and evaluation, the model may be used to guide practice and education by providing a structure

Table 2 Guided Care Model: Illustration of the Relationship between
Care Coordination Interventions, Process Goals, and Outcomes

Care Coordination Interventions	Process Goals	Care Coordination Outcomes (examples)
Monitoring and Coaching	85% of patients have contact each month for monitoring and coaching	Physical & Mental Health Quality of Life Patient Satisfaction
Caregiver Support	At least 75% of caregivers are contacted once every three months	Caregiver satisfation Caregiver strain
Education on Advance Directives	100% of patients have written advance directives	Service use Patient and family Satisfaction
Communication with Members of Healthcare Team	Contact with each team member every two months	Medication adherence Provider satisfaction
Transitional Care	100% of hospitalized patients are visited within two days of admissions 100% of hospitalized patients are seen at home within two days of discharge	Reduction in hospital readmissions Reduction in hospital costs

to develop RN competencies and teaching materials for care coordination and transition management beyond the hospital walls.

Logic models have long been used in program evaluation. They specify relationships among program goals, objectives, activities, outputs, and outcomes. They indicate the theoretical connections between program components, activities involved, and individuals responsible for carrying out the activities and specification of short-, medium-, and long-term outcomes. In addition, logic models used for evaluation include the measures that will be used to determine if activities were carried out as planned (process and output measures) and if the program's objectives have been met (outcome measures) (BJA CPEPM, 2013).

The RN-Care Coordination Transition Management (RN-CCTM) Logic Model (Table 3) was developed to clearly explicate the dimensions/competencies of RN care coordination and transition management in ambulatory care, specific care coordination activities, and providers involved, as well as the short-, medium-, and long-term outcomes. Using this model makes it possible to incorporate measures of care coordination and transition management dimensions, processes, and outcomes so that the causal relationships can be traced and analyzed. When measures or indicators are embedded in routine electronic documentation and standardized language coding is used, the

Table 3 RN-CCTM Model Logic Model

Inputs/ Competencies	Outputs		Outcomes		
	Activities →	Participation →	Short →	Medium →	Long
Support for self management	Enhance health literacy	RN-CCTM, MD, APRN, pharmacist, social worker	Baseline comprehensive needs assessment reflects patient values, preferences, goals	Solutions to most critical socioeconomic issues	Engaged, educated patient/family, increased ability to "cope" with care interventions
Advocacy	Negotiate and secure patient services Coach patient in self advocacy	RN-CCTM, MD, APRN, pharmacist, social worker	Patient/family concerns and goals heard, able to access providers, community services, medications	Patient/family compliance with treatment plan, medications	Keep primary care appointments, appointments in community agencies
Education and engagement of patient and family	Assess readiness to learn/learning styles	RN-CCTM, pharmacist, social worker, dietician, psychologist	Patient/family can "teach back" info on care interventions	Increased engagement in preventative care and use of telehealth learning modalities	Engaged, educated patient/family
Cross setting communication and transition	Coordination/collaboration between specialty and primary providers who use the Patient Care Plan across settings	RN-CCTM, MD, APRN, pharmacist, social worker, dietician, psychologist, MD specialists, acute care, LTC, and home care RNs	Patient Care Plan transmitted between setting, changes and updates communicated	Use of electronic Patient Care Plan for handoffs	Decreased errors, duplication, costs
Coaching and counseling of patients and families	Answer questions patients/families have before and after seeing provider visit	RN-CCTM	Patients/families come prepared with "Ask Me Three" questions to clinic or calls	Enhanced understanding of healthcare resources in the community and the need to seek consultation prior to increased severity	Decreased ED use Increased ability to "cope" with care interventions
Nursing process	Assess patient for knowledge understanding diagnosis, needs, Rx, expected outcomes of Rx	RN-CCTM	Best evidence used for interventions/outcomes Patient Care Plan is routinely updated	Electronic process indicators show compliance with EBP plan, short term EBP outcomes achieved	Long term EBP disease or health outcomes achieved at 80% level
Population health management	Expert use of population management tools (e.g. registries, analytics tools) to track and monitor select population characteristics	RN-CCTM, MD, APRN, Pharmacist, social worker, dietician, MA, psychologist, MD specialists, acute care, LTC, and home care RNs	Maximize impact of visit or telehealth call regarding disease management, prevention, and wellness through alerts	Enhanced process improvement, enhanced immunization rates, and participation in wellness programming	Enhanced quality of care, achievement of benchmarks for prevention and wellness

Table 3 RN-CCTM Model Logic Model

Inputs/ Competencies	Outputs		Outcomes		
	Activities →	Participation →	Short →	Medium →	Long
Team work and collaboration	Inclusion of team-work in orientation and CE	RN-CCTM, MD, APRN, pharmacist, social worker, dietician, MA, psychologist, MD specialists, acute care, LTC, and home care RNs	Enhanced under-standing of inter-disciplinary roles and communica-tion techniques	Early collaboration when issue arises, team problem solving/planning	Less siloed care Engaged health-care team Increased appreciation of team member contributions
Patient-centered care planning	Motivational inter-viewing, eliciting patient's goals and priorities	RN-CCTM, MD, APRN, Pharmacist, social worker, dietician, MA, psychologist, MD specialists, acute care, LTC, and home care RNs	Individualized Care Plan Care planning activities transcend barriers/ transitions keeping the patient at the focus	Plan of care transparent for patient/family and perceive team is listening to their preferences/goals	Enhanced patient/ family engage-ment and satisfac-tion with quality of care

Situation: The Registered Nurse-Care Coordination Transition Management (RN-CCTM) Logic Model evolved to standard-ize work of ambulatory care nurses using evidence from interdisciplinary literature on care coordination and transition man-agement. The vision is the RN-CCTM Model would specify dimensions of CCTM and competencies needed to perform CCTM and make possible development of knowledge, skills, and attitudes needed for each competency so the RN-CCTM will meet needs of patients with complex chronic illnesses being cared for in patient-centered medical homes (PCMH) and their preparation and work as an RN-CCTM would be recognized by a certificate credential from the American Nurses Credentialing Center (ANCC) and reimbursed by CMS.

Assumptions: Patients will use primary care settings, patients will access RN-CCTM providers. Patients will be engaged in care processes. Providers will collaborate, work in teams, develop and use patient-centered care plans. Organization will have EHR that operates across settings. Outcomes are shared by team, not discipline-specific

External Factors: Slow development of interdisciplinary team education and practice. Changes in reimbursement and penalties for never events are decreasing revenues, slow implementation of EMRs that are operable across settings, and slow development of model for care plan that moves between settings.

electronic health record documentation can be queried to determine compliance with processes and the outcomes achieved.

The RN-CCTM Logic Model also includes contextual factors that may affect whether care coordination interventions result in expected outcomes. For instance, patient beliefs about primary care and emergency room services may override the best efforts to reduce emergency room use. For example, a recent study by Kangovi and colleagues (2013) found that chronically ill patients with Medicaid coverage chose to go to an emergency room because they found the care there more convenient, higher quality, and less expen-sive to them than their primary care setting. Their determination of convenience was influenced by current Medicaid rules that do not support requests for transportation for same day access to primary care. They expressed the belief that there was higher quality care in the ED and that they could be seen by specialists in one visit rather than having to take time off from work to see specialists that they are referred to from primary care. Patient interviews revealed telling statements such as "The [primary care doctor] never treated me or my husband aggressively to get blood pressure under control. I went to the hospital and they had it under control in four days. The [physician] had three years." (Kangovi et al., 2013, p. 1198). Out-of-pocket costs for the emergency room visit were lower than their primary care visits which were associated with a co-payment at the time of the visit. Although the study sample size was small, this study yielded provocative findings about the importance of contextual factors that frequently are not measured, or considered, when examining the relationship between care coordination interventions and outcomes. Changing these patients' use of emergency room visits would need to take the factors of perceptions of convenience, quality, and cost into account.

The RN-CCTM Logic Model shown in Table 3 is condensed for this chapter and is intended to demonstrate how such a model can be used. Each competency or input in the first column of the model is followed by care coordination activities, the responsible person, and short-, medium-, and long-term outcomes. The model identifies who is accountable for documentation within each competency area and the content for documentation, such as patient/family concerns and goals in the individualized care plan. Indicators for short- and medium-term outcomes may be developed and embedded in routine electronic documentation and provide a process trail for tracking long-term outcome measures.

Measurement of Care Coordination Processes and Selected Outcomes

Quality of care for individuals with complex healthcare needs often is unintentionally fragmented and unsafe. The story of Catherine Jenkins (see sidebar on next page) describes a common patient experience and emphasizes the need for measuring and improving care coordination. Examples are provided to illustrate how the RN-CCTM Logic Model may be used to guide these efforts.

As described in the RN-CCTM Model, support for self-management commences with inputs/competencies, such as use of a validated assessment tool to determine patient needs, be they socioeconomic, physical, psychosocial, or health needs. This assessment also includes elicitation of patient values, preferences, and goals. The RN communicates findings to patient-centered medical home (PCMH) team members and works collaboratively with social workers to obtain needed referrals, access for services, and to communicate via the electronic care plan the patient/family's values, preferences, and goals. The logic model then specifies some of the short-, medium-, and long-term outcomes of

Using the RN-CC Logic Model to Guide Care Coordination Interventions and Measurement

Catherine Jenkins is a 70-year-old retired high school guidance counselor. She is single and lives alone in her home with her dog. She receives social security checks, a small pension, and Medicare with basic coverage for medication. She has a son who is married with two teenage daughters, and lives about 25 miles away. Ms. Jenkins has four chronic conditions: hypertension, diabetes, heart failure, and rheumatoid arthritis. She sees six different physicians for these conditions and takes eight medications.

In 2012, Ms. Jenkins had a difficult year. She had several exacerbations of her conditions, including four hospitalizations for her heart failure and hypertension. Her diabetes became less controlled and she has increased pain due to her rheumatoid arthritis. She spent time in two nursing homes and received home care from two different agencies. She was referred to six different community agencies for assistance at home.

Ms. Jenkins is confused about her medications. She does not understand her diabetic diet and does not monitor her blood pressure. She describes her quality of life as poor. Her son dreads calls from her, as well as the many providers and agencies involved in her care. He has no idea what to do about all the bills, the different doctors, and the different appointments. At this point, he is ready to put his mother in a nursing home. He cannot handle managing her care and is fearful for her safety.

This is a common story that is told by many individuals and their families across the nation. How can you use the RN-CCTM model to guide you in developing, measuring, and evaluating a coordinated care plan for Ms. Jenkins and her family?

1. What care coordination activities/competencies are needed?

2. Who is the most appropriate person or professional to implement these activities?

3. What are the priorities for short-, moderate-, and long-term outcomes?

the assessment, collaboration, and beginning development of the electronic individualized care plan.

Medication Management

Medication management is linked to the nursing process, where assessment of patient/family understanding of prescribed medications, dosage, when and why they are needed, how they work, and what potential side effects to look for are emphasized. The RN would employ evidence-based interventions such as "teach back" to enhance patient/family understanding of medications while reinforcing the patient role in decision-making regarding medications. The RN would communicate with the pharmacist and providers regarding medication issues and work with them and the family to come up with solutions. Solutions would be communicated on the electronic individualized care plan both within and beyond the hospital walls and would also help to extend the reach of the interprofessional care team post-discharge. Again, the logic model specifies some of the short-, medium-, and long-term outcomes of the assessment, collaboration, and use of the electronic individualized care plan.

Safe Practices

Safe practices have been a focus of healthcare delivery from many perspectives and have assumed more prominence with the ACA provisions fostering prevention. Safe practices may include care coordination activities linked to population health management and would include interventions across the continuum, such as immunizations alerts so immunizations are given in a timely manner. Safe practices may also include coaching and counseling to stress safe practices in the home to prevent falls, pressure ulcers, and infections. Foundational to ensuring safe practices is identifying a clear strategy and continuously reinforcing the necessary activities for effective safe practice.

Implications for Practice, Education, and Research

Earlier in this chapter, several care coordination interventions were discussed including patient engagement and self-care practices, medication management, safe practices, and prevention of healthcare-acquired conditions. When issues such as these are discussed without consideration to how they work with the routine work processes of healthcare providers, the preparation needed for providers to be competent in interventions to prevent or deal with these issues, and evaluation strategies to determine if objectives are met, they may not get the consistency of attention and follow through needed. Also, if not provided the thorough attention required, these issues will persist and continue

Table 4 Selected Safe Practices Related to Care Coordination and Associated Outcomes

NQF	AHRQ	Outcomes
Teamwork Training and Skill Building		Reduce preventable harm
Identification and Mitigation of Risks and Hazards	Routine Surveillance for Prevention of Healthcare-Associated Infections Patient Safety Practices Targeted at Diagnostic Error Monitoring Patient Safety Problems	Reduce preventable harm
Informed Consent		Verbalize understanding
Nursing Workforce		Reinforce patient safeguards
Patient Care Information	Promoting Engagement by Patients and Families to Reduce Adverse Events	Provide information necessary for continued care
Discharge Systems	Interventions to Improve Care Transitions at Hospital Discharge	Provide information necessary for continued care Reduce readmissions
Medication Reconciliation	Medication Reconciliation	Provide information necessary for continued care Reduce medication errors Reduce adverse drug reactions
Fall Prevention		Reduce falls across care continuum Reduce fall-related injuries across care continuum

to engender poor quality of care and outcomes. If we are to achieve quality and safety outcomes across the healthcare continuum, what is needed is an evidence-based role for healthcare providers that is responsive to expectations of care spelled out in the ACA (2010) and that incorporates all of the major dimensions of care coordination and transition management.

Providers must be prepared and competent in all of the interventions involved in each dimension of care coordination. As noted in many of the earlier chapters, establishing strong support for the relationships between care coordination and transition management interventions and quality and safety outcomes relies on clear explication and measurement of the processes and short-, medium-, and long-term outcomes of such care. This is necessary not only to educate providers, but also to develop and implement measures of adherence to evidence-based processes and outcomes. Such evaluation is critical to ongoing refinement of interventions and monitoring of outcomes. National reports have called for patient-centric care models as one strategy to improve the quality of care (IOM, 2001). A 2010 Institute of Medicine (IOM) report, *The Future of Nursing*, again reiterated this call for patient-centered care and identified the need to reconsider the roles of health professionals, including RNs, and transform practices related to care coordination.

Research findings indicate that care coordination may exert its influence through relationship building and a focus on patient-centered care. An early national study of the RN role in ambulatory care identified long-term patient and family relationships as a significant reason that nurses remained in ambulatory care and that care coordination is a major dimension of the overall professional nurse's role (Haas & Hackbarth, 1995; Haas, Hackbarth, Kavanaugh, & Vlasses, 1995). The provisions of the 2010 Affordable Care Act called for care coordination and evidence-based practice, but the law does not spell out who should do it or how it should be done. Leaders in ambulatory care have long known that nurses do care coordination and transition management, but it is not clearly spelled out as a part of their role and rarely are there electronic documentation formats that allow documentation on care coordination or transition management done by nurses. Thus, as described in Chapter 5, there is little evidence of this work by nurses in ambulatory care settings.

Recently, the Affordable Care Act was the impetus to formalize the role of the ambulatory care RN in care coordination and transition management. With the renewed support of the patient-centered medical home (PCMH) model, there was widespread recognition of the importance and opportunity for nurses in primary care and ambulatory settings to deliver core care coordination and transition management interventions. The American Academy of Ambulatory Care Nursing (AAACN), the national organization of nurses working in ambulatory care settings, implemented a task force to develop and execute a care coordination competencies action plan that would provide a blueprint for assisting RNs to take on care coordination roles and demonstrate their effectiveness. The action plan is being carried out in four phases and is described here in some depth to demonstrate the active role nurses and professional organizations are taking to advance nurse care coordination in all settings. It is important to note the systematic and strong evidence-based foundation for this care coordination action plan.

- Phase 1: Analyze the interdisciplinary evidence on care coordination and transition management
- Phase 2: Delineate ambulatory RN dimensions and competencies

- Phase 3: Develop an RN care coordination and transition management model
- Phase 4: Develop an education program for an RN role in care coordination and transition management within the healthcare team in ambulatory care and the PCMH

Volunteer expert panels consisting of ambulatory nurses using focus group methods online participated in all phases of this project. Following a search in MEDLINE, CINAHL Plus, and PsycINFO, the first 26-member expert panel worked in dyads and analyzed 82 interdisciplinary journal articles and abstracted data to a table of evidence (TOE) (Haas, Swan, & Haynes, 2013). The TOE included designation of those materials that discussed care coordination and transition management dimensions of care.

Phase 2 expert panelists developed competencies for care coordination and transition management dimensions guided by the Quality and Safety Education in Nursing (QSEN) method of indicating knowledge, skills, and attitudes requisite to each dimension (Cronenwett et al., 2007). The expert panelists represented diverse practice and education experience: public, private, military, and veterans organizations, and 15 states in the east, west, north, south, and central United States plus the District of Columbia. Nine dimensions of care coordination and transition management were identified and are shown in Table 5.

Phase 3 expert panelists were guided in their deliberations by the Wagner Chronic Care Model (1998). They reviewed, confirmed, and finalized a table of dimensions, competencies (including knowledge, skills, and attitudes), and activities for ambulatory care RN care coordination and transition management. After much discussion, the third expert panel further determined that the original eighth dimension of decision support

Table 5 Nine Dimensions of Care Coordination and Transition Management for Ambulatory Care Nursing

- Support for self-management
- Education and engagement of patient and family
- Cross setting communication and transition
- Coaching and counseling of patients and families
- Nursing process including assessment, plan, implementation/intervention, and evaluation, a proxy for monitoring and intervening
- Team work and collaboration
- Patient-centered care planning
- Population health management
- Advocacy

Source: Adapted from Haas, Swan, & Haynes, 2013

and information systems, as well as telehealth practice, were technologies that support all care coordination. Thus, transition management dimensions and population health management became the new eighth dimension given the prominence it is assuming in outpatient care even though there was little discussion of it in the extant literature and activities for ambulatory care RN care coordination and transition management. This expert panel also determined methods to be used to enhance teamwork and interprofessional collaboration in outpatient settings. Nationally recognized core competencies for interprofessional collaborative practice (AACN, 2011), quality and safety in nursing education (QSEN) competencies (Cronenwett et al., 2007), and public health nursing competencies (Quad Council, 2011) overlap with the dimensions and competencies needed for ambulatory care RN care coordination and transition management.

Phase 4 expert panelists are developing structured education modules for each dimension and producing a RN Care Coordination and Transition Management Core Curriculum text and webinars to support development of RNs in ambulatory care settings to fulfill the RN-CCTM role. This is only one of many exciting and important examples of national initiatives to prepare nurses for important new care coordination opportunities.

CONCLUSION

Modeling of processes and outcomes is challenging but necessary if we hope to determine and track best practices' processes and outcomes. The RN-CCTM Logic Model recognizes that many of the dimensions of care coordination and transition management are not exclusively the domain of nurses. It accentuates the importance of demonstrating how nurses function as a part of an interprofessional team and the value they add to the work of the team. This is especially needed in ambulatory care where the work and value of nurses is largely invisible. Consequently, work must be done to define the RN's role in care coordination and transition management, educate nurses to develop competencies needed to perform in this area, and work with administration and vendors to develop documentation screens that reflect the dimensions, activities, processes/outputs, and outcomes that RNs accomplish with patients in ambulatory settings. Mining data generated from such documentation in the electronic record will ultimately demonstrate the value of nurses as part of the interprofessional team.

Another important challenge is to develop process and outcome measures that reflect nurses' contribution to care coordination and transition management. The American Nurses Association (ANA) has responded to this challenge with the creation of a Care Coordination Quality Measurement Panel Steering Committee (ANA, 2013) composed of national experts in this area and representing major specialty nursing organizations. Thus far, this panel has built a framework for exploration and development of measures. When complete, this framework will be a stimulus and guide for measure development and testing. There is a need to move beyond the use of easily accessed outcomes to more discrete outcome measures that are linked to intervention processes. This allows evidence-based processes to be defined and promulgated as we work to enhance quality and safety outcomes from care coordination and transition management.

Finally, given the diversity in approaches being developed in accountable care organizations (ACOs) and PCMHs, there are opportunities for many care coordination and transition management models to be developed, tested, and modified to meet the unique needs of patient populations served. When electronic patient records are fully operationalized across the care continuum and all members of the interprofessional team are documenting in them, we will have a rich repository of real-time data that will further inform development of delivery models that enhance safety, quality, and cost-effective care for patients.

REFERENCES

Agency for Healthcare Research and Quality (AHRQ). (2011). National strategy for quality improvement in health care. Report to Congress.

Agency for Healthcare Research and Quality (AHRQ). (2012a). Coordinating care for adults with complex care needs in the patient-centered medical home: Challenges and solutions. Retrieved from http://pcmh.ahrq.gov/portal/server.pt/community/pcmh__home/1483/

Agency for Healthcare Research and Quality (AHRQ). (2012b). Medication adherence interventions: Comparative effectiveness. Rockville, MD: AHRQ Publication No. 12-E010-1.

Agency for Healthcare Research and Quality (AHRQ). (2013a). Closing the quality gap: Revisiting the state of the science. Rockville, MD: AHRQ Publication No. 12(13)-E017.

Agency for Healthcare Research and Quality (AHRQ). (2013b). Making health care safer II. Rockville, MD: AHRQ Publication No. 13-E001-EF

Aliotta, S., Grieve, K., Giddens, J., Dunbar, L., Groves, C., Frey, K., & Boult, C. (2008). Guided care: A new frontier for adults with chronic conditions. *Professional Care Management, 13*(3), 151–158.

American Association of Colleges of Nursing. (AACN). (2011). Core competencies for interprofessional collaborative practice. Retrieved from http://www.aacn.nche.edu/education-resources/ipecreport.pdf

American Nursing Association (ANA). (2013). Care coordination quality measurement panel steering committee. Retrieved from http://www.nursingworld.org/MainMenuCategories/Policy-Advocacy/Professional-Issues-Panels/Care-Coordination-Quality-Measures-Panel

Boult, C., Karm, L., & Groves, C. (2008). Improving chronic care: The "Guided Care" model. *The Permanente Journal, 12*(1), 50–54.

Boyd, C., Boult, C., Shadmi, E., Leff, B., Brager, R., Dunbar, L., ... Wegener, S. (2007). Guided care for multimorbid older adults. *The Gerontologist, 47*(5), 697–704

Bureau of Justice Assistance Center for Program Evaluation and Performance Measurement (BJA CPEPM). (2013). Planning the evaluation: Developing and working with program logic models. Retrieved from https://www.bja.gov/evaluation/guide/pe4.htm

Coburn, K. D., Marcantonio S., Lazansky R., Keller, M., & Davis, N. (2012). Effect of a community-based nursing intervention on mortality in chronically ill older adults: A randomized controlled trial. *PLOS Medicine, 9*(7), e1001265. doi:10.1371/journal.pmed.1001265

Craig, C., Eby, D., & Whittington, J. (2011). *Care coordination model: Better care at lower cost for people with multiple health and social needs.* IHI Innovation Series white paper. Cambridge, MA: Institute for Healthcare Improvement. Retrieved from http://www.ihi.org/knowledge/Pages/IHIWhitePapers/IHICareCoordinationModelWhitePaper.aspx

Cronenwett, L., Sherwood, G., Barnsteiner, J., Disch, J., Johnson, J., Mitchell, P., ... Warren, J. (2007). Quality and safety education for nurses. *Nursing Outlook, 55*(3), 122–131.

Haas, S., Hackbarth, D., Kavanagh, J., & Vlasses, F. (1995). Dimensions of the staff nurse role in ambulatory care: Part II—Comparison of role dimensions in four ambulatory settings. *Nursing Economic$, 13*(3), 152–165.

Haas, S., & Hackbarth, D. (1995). Dimensions of the staff nurse role in ambulatory care: Part III—Using research data to design new models of nursing care delivery. *Nursing Economic$, 13*(4), 230–241.

Haas, S., Swan, B. A., & Haynes, T. (2013). Developing ambulatory care registered nurse competencies for care coordination and transition management. *Nursing Economic$, 31*(1), 41–48.

Hibbard, J., & Greene, J. (2013). What the evidence shows about patient activation: Better health outcomes and care experiences; fewer data on costs. *Health Affairs, 32*(2), 207–214.

Institute of Medicine (IOM). (2001). *Crossing the quality chasm: A new health system for the 21st century.* Washington D.C.: National Academies Press.

Institute of Medicine (IOM). (2010). *The future of nursing: Leading change, advancing health.* (1st ed.). Washington D.C.: National Academies Press.

Kangovi, S., Barg, F., Carter, T., Long, J., Shannon, R., & Grande, D. (2013). Understanding why patients of low socioeconomic status prefer hospitals over ambulatory care. *Health Affairs, 32*(7), 1196–1203.

National Quality Forum (NQF). (2013). *National quality forum endorsed set of 34 safe practices.* Washington, D.C.: Author.

Quad Council. (2011). Quad council public health nursing competencies. Retrieved from http://www.phf.org/resourcestools/Pages/Public_Health_Nursing_Competencies.aspx

Swan, B. A. (2012). A nurse learns firsthand that you may fend for yourself after a hospital stay. *Health   Affairs, 31*(11), 2579–2582.

Wagner, E. H. (1998). Chronic disease management: What will it take to improve care for chronic illness? *Effective Clinical Practice, 1*(1), 2–4.

ACKNOWLEDGEMENTS

The authors wish to recognize the members of the AACN Care Coordination Transitional Care Management Expert Panel including Karen Alexander, MSN, RN, CCRN; Janine Allbritton, BSN, RN; JoAnn Appleyard, PhD, RN; Jill Arzouman, MS, RN, ACNS, BC, CMSRN; Deborah Aylard, MSN, RN; Deanna Blanchard, MSN, RN; Elizabeth Bradley, MSN, RN-BC; Stefanie Coffey, DNP, MBA, FNP-BC, RN-BC; Sandy Fights, MS, RN, CMSRN, CNE; Jan Fuch, MBS, MSN, NEA-BC; Patricia Grady, BSN, RN, CRNS, FABC; Jamie Green, MSN, RN; Denise Hannagan, MSN, MHA, RN-BC; Clare Hastings, PhD, RN, FAAN; Anne Jessie, MSN, RN; Sheila Johnson, MBA, RN; Diane Kelly, DrPH, MBA, RN; Lisa Kristosik, MSN, RN; Cheryl Lovlien, MS, RN-BC; Rosemarie Marmion, MSN, RN-BC, NE-BC; Nancy May, MSN, BSN, RN-BC; Sylvia McKenzie, MSN, RN, CPHQ, CDR; Catherine McNeal Jones, MBA, HCM, RN BC; Kathy Mertens, MN, MPH, RN; Shirley Morrison, PhD, RN, OCN; Janet Moye, PhD, RN, NEA-BC; Donna Parker, MA, BSN, RN-BC; Carol Rutenberg, MNSc, RN-BC, C-TNP; Deborah Smith, DNP, RN; Debra Toney, PhD, RN, FAAN; Barbara Trehearne, PhD, RN; Linda Walton, MSN, RN, CRNP; and Stephanie Witwer, PhD, RN, NEA-BC.

Chapter 9

Care Coordination and Health Information Technology

Rosemary Kennedy, PhD, RN, MBA, FAAN; Patricia S. Button, EdD, RN; Patricia C. Dykes, PhD, RN, FAAN, FACMI; Laura K. Heerman Langford, PhD, RN; and Lipika Samal, MD, MPH

Health information technology (HIT) is a necessary requirement for high quality, safe, and effective care coordination. Irrespective of the various models and methods of care coordination, all require effective communication and decision-making across care settings, providers, and receivers of care. Furthermore, with advent of the health care home, the setting of care coordination is frequently the home, community, school, and workplace, requiring ubiquitous information exchange.

HIT can support the activities related to care coordination, facilitate transfer of information, enable communication between parties in different locations, and provide real-time decision support. HIT can reduce unnecessary and costly duplication of services by sharing service results across settings of care. The electronic health record (EHR) can prevent medication errors by informing clinicians of patient allergies, providing patient education information, and reconciling medication lists as patients move from one setting of care to another (Congressional Budget Office, 2008). Care coordination models vary, but typically, they utilize case managers, care transition programs, disease management, HIT, and other strategies to manage service delivery and support patients and providers. Care coordination combined with the use of HIT has the potential to reduce cost and improve outcomes for all populations in all health care settings; the most impressive outcomes occur in high-risk populations whose complex health issues involve costly treatments and repeated hospitalizations (NQF, 2010). The purpose of this chapter is to describe the rapidly evolving role of HIT in advancing the goals of care coordination, and to propose strategies for nurses and other professionals to anticipate and influence future developments in the field.

DEFINITION OF HIT TERMS

HIT, as an important component in care coordination, is the application of computers and technology to the provision of healthcare in all settings, including all stakeholders involved in health (Hersch, 2009). Since HIT plays a critical role in communication, frequently the term information and communications technology (ICT) is used along with HIT. There are different technologies that are included under the umbrella term of HIT. One of national importance is the EHR, which includes comprehensive and longitudinal information about the patient's supporting care across all settings (acute, home-care, ambulatory, clinic, etc.). The Healthcare Information and Management Systems Society (HIMSS) define EHR as a secure, real-time, point-of-care, patient-centric information resource for clinicians (HIMSS, 2003). The EHR ideally facilitates care coordination by providing ubiquitous access to information and evidence-based alerts and reminders across people, function, and sites over time. HIT plays a key role in the major domains of care coordination as defined by the National Quality Forum (NQF), including the health care home, creation of a proactive plan of care, and follow-up, communication, and transition of care or hand-off support (NQF, 2006).

The EHR automates and streamlines care coordination workflow, closing gaps in communication and responses that can cause delays in care. EHRs are typically tailored for the specific needs of a respective facility and the operations of that facility. Therefore, in order to support care coordination between and among facilities, health information exchanges (HIEs) are needed. Linking all of the HIT systems within a region or community is essential in order to exchange important health information across different EHRs spanning different healthcare delivery organizations. HIEs enable the digital exchange of health information across organizations within a region or community of care (Alliance for Health Reform, n.d.).

Personal health records (PHRs) store healthcare information that is entered and managed by the patient and/or consumer of health care (HealthIT.gov, n.d.-a.). PHRs typically contain patient reported care compliance, clinical status, and outcome information that is critical data for effective care coordination. Patient access to the information in their electronic health records is very important and with patient portals, patients have secure, online, 24-hour access to personal health information, such as medications, laboratory results, and care plans, from any location through the Internet (HealthIT. gov, n.d.-b). The data contained within EHRs and PHRs can be downloaded onto mobile technology platforms, such as iPads and smartphones. This facilitates exchange of information between not only nurses, physicians, and care team members, but also the patients, thereby making them part of the care team. Care coordination requires HIT that supports on-demand access to information, on any device (phone, laptop, tablets, workstations), serving multiple users at once (nurse, physician, patient, consumer), and using technology so the users do not have to be concerned about where the information is stored. This is the essence of cloud computing. The major advantage of cloud computing for care coordination is "on demand" access to information without requiring human interaction with individual service providers. The advent of cloud computing allows for ubiquitous, convenient, on-demand network access to a pool of applications, servers, and services that can be accessed with minimal effort (Mell & Grance, 2011). With the appropriate security and patient privacy software, cloud computing can be a tool to facilitate information exchange across geographical settings, providers, and patients.

Also, the Internet serves as a valuable source of education information that can be used to support care coordination activities, particularly when patients move from one setting of care to another. As nurses advise and educate patients, it is important to assess the Internet sources of education using criteria ensuring the entity posting the information is a valid and reliable source of evidence-based content, that original sources of publication are provided, and that the information is reviewed by someone with the appropriate credentials before it is posted (National Cancer Institute, 2012).

The science that goes into HIT focuses on the specialty of informatics. As defined by the Nursing Informatics (NI) Special Interest Group of the International Medical Informatics Association (IMIA), nursing informatics science and practice "integrates nursing, its information and knowledge, and their management with information and communication technologies to promote the health of people, families, and communities world-wide" (IMIA News, 2009, paragraph 2).

THE ROLE OF HIT IN CARE COORDINATION

The National Quality Strategy's (NQS) aims of better care, affordable care, and healthy people and communities set forth a unified vision of the healthcare system (NQS, 2012). In 2011, the NQS focused national attention on care coordination, aligning efforts on the use of HIT to focus on effective communication to coordinate care. Integral to these efforts is the use of HIT to capture, aggregate, and report data to enable more standardized and efficient care delivery at both the patient and population level.

The use of HIT is important to the NQS and, to this extent, the Health Information Technology for Economic and Clinical Health Act of 2009 fosters adoption of meaningful use (MU) of certified EHRs to improve quality and reduce healthcare costs through financial incentives (Harle, Huerta, Ford, Diana, & Menachemi, 2013). This has significant implications for care coordination, as MU requires the exchange of electronic health information with other systems and to also integrate the information into care delivery (U.S. Government Printing Office, 2009). The exchange of information within and between sources of care, whether HIT or providers of care, is an integral function of care coordination; therefore, the MU requirements are aligned to support care coordination activities.

Concurrently, the Agency for Healthcare Research and Quality's (AHRQ) care coordination framework diagrams key domains that are important for care coordination (AHRQ, 2011), while also providing a mechanism for describing the use of HIT. The AHRQ framework identifies coordination activities hypothesized or demonstrated to facilitate both the care coordination activities and the broad approaches that are commonly used to improve the delivery of health care, including improving care coordination. This framework identifies "health IT-enabled coordination" as a broad approach to support coordination (AHRQ, 2011). Health IT tools, such as EHRs, patient portals, or databases, can be used to communicate information about patients and their care between healthcare entities or to maintain information over time. Table 1 shows the components of the framework along with examples of how HIT supports the framework.

Table 1 AHRQ Mechanisms for Achieving Care
Coordination (Domains) with HIT Examples

Coordination Activities	HIT Examples
Establish accountability or negotiate responsibility	■ Electronic tracking of patient consent forms across settings of care. ■ Worklists showing all members of the clinical team and respective areas of responsibility to facilitate patient understanding as they transition from acute care to home care.
Communicate	■ Patient access to a plan of care that displays reminders for medications. ■ Patient entry of reported outcomes (blood pressure, blood sugars) into smartphones that automatically alert the nurse in the clinic if the result is out of range for real-time communication between patient and provider.
Facilitate transitions	■ Seamless and secure exchange of patient summary information between the acute care nurse and the home care nurse to support transitions of care. ■ Home case nurse has electronic access to the patient care plan prior to hospital discharge to allow for care coordination and management.
Assess needs and goals	■ Evidence-based suggested problem list based on nurse documentation of an admission assessment. ■ Integration of data entered into a PHR with data entered into an EHR so a nurse can develop a person-centered care plan in accordance with patient preferences.

Coordination Activities	HIT Examples
Create a proactive plan of care	■ Use of clinical decision support to create a proactive plan of care based on assessment documentation from all members of the clinical team.
Monitor, follow-up, and respond to change	■ Use of electronic alerts so when a physical therapist visits a home care patient and identifies a high fall risk score, an alert is sent to the home care nurse for immediate follow-up.
Support self-management goals	■ Integration of patient documented goals (from a PHR) into the EHR to provide a comprehensive list to the home care nurse before the first home care visit.
Link to community resources	■ Easy access from the EHR to community resources that fit the patient's needs based on data entered into the EHR (diagnoses, conditions, age, etc.).
Align resources with patient and population needs	■ Transmission of patient data to home care nurses prior to discharge for appropriate alignment between patient needs and nurse expertise.
	■ Electronic systems can determine where failures in care are occurring by mining large databases to determine which nursing interventions have the highest impact on outcomes across populations.
Broad Approaches	HIT Examples
Teamwork focused on coordination	■ Use of a clinical summary seamlessly transmitted between physician provider, home care nurse, and pharmacist for care coordination in the community so all stakeholders have access to the most up-to-date information. See Case 4.
Health care home	■ Real-time communication of pertinent home care nurse documentation to the physician provider prior to the initial office visit after a hospital discharge.
Care management	■ Engaging patients in use of technology to enter patient reported outcomes, receive reminders related to medications, and with real time communication to providers if patients are not following the care plan. See Case 2.
Medication management	■ Patient entry of actual medication use through interactive phone voice technology that feeds a dashboard for early intervention by a nurse if the medication is not being followed as ordered. See Case 3.
Health IT-enabled care coordination	■ Use of health information exchanges whereby patient information is securely communicated between providers using disparate EHR systems. This facilitates care coordination when a patient receiving care from one system is admitted to a facility in another system. The HIE ensures that nurses have access to all the patient information. See Cases 1 and 5.

Source: Domains (left column) from AHRQ, 2011

Essential national efforts underway are fostering the development and implementation of HIT to support care coordination with the intent to increase quality, safety, and effectiveness. HIT enabled care coordination includes:

- Development and adoption of databases that store important information related to nursing practice (evidence-based care plans), patient specific information (assessment findings, medications, laboratory results), financial information (insurance data), and administrative information (past visits, locations, and providers). All of this information is vital to care coordination as the database can support an episode of care, as well as transitions of care between acute and home care settings.

- Software applications that provide the functionality necessary to view patient data, enter patient data, generate reports, and communicate with both the patient and the interprofessional team.

- Clinical decision support tools that foster decision-making based on current research and best practices, as well as providing the ability to assess the impact of nursing care across patient populations, ultimately generating new knowledge to advance nursing practice.

- Development and adoption of data standards starting with the use of a consistent standardized terminology, which serves as the infrastructure behind the use of HIT for care coordination. Consistent use of terms for concepts (pressure ulcers, pain, etc.) is critical for the exchange of data between disparate HIT systems across geographical settings. If the systems use different terms, it will be extremely arduous trying to send data between the hospital system and the home care system. Without this consistent representation using standard codes, nurses will have to interpret the data between different systems, thereby hindering efficiency, quality, and safety.

HIT IN CARE COORDINATION: SOME CASE EXAMPLES

In the previous section, we discussed HIT solutions that could support effective care coordination and care transitions within settings and across the continuum. Consider the following cases and how lack of information can lead to suboptimal outcomes. Also consider how information exchanges might differ in primary care, hospital, or post-acute settings and how this will influence effective care coordination.

Case 1. Pediatric Care

An eight-year-old child cared for by a PCP in the community has frequent admissions to an acute care hospital for a pulmonary condition. While on vacation, the child becomes acutely short of breath and the family takes him to a local ED. The ED has no information on the child's chronic medical condition and the child is given nebulizers with no improvement. The child is admitted to a general pediatrics unit in the hospital. The inpatient team does not have access to a current problem list, a current list of outpatient meds, or an emergency care plan. They gather information from the family about the patient's condition and medications, but the information is not specific enough to assist in diagnosis and treatment of the acute exacerbation. The patient's specialist is not reachable by phone. Fortunately, the child does not need to be intubated overnight and the inpatient team receives a call back from the specialist the following morning, at which time a recent note is faxed over that helps the inpatient team to diagnose and treat the patient.

- How would a health information exchange have improved care transitions for this patient?

- What health information technologies could be used to enhance follow-up care and greater engagement of the child and family in self-care?

Case 2. Acute Care

A 76-year-old patient with heart failure is brought by ambulance to an ED at a community hospital after being seen there and discharged one week ago with medication changes and a recommendation to follow-up with the primary care provider. The patient presents with a weight gain of seven pounds, shortness of breath, and fatigue. The patient gives a medication list to the ED nurse that was prepared three months earlier by the visiting nurse. The medication list is not reconciled to reflect the changes from the previous ED visit. The patient says that he did not follow-up with his primary care provider because he was feeling too weak to leave the house. The patient reports that he has several self-management plans: one from the ED, another from the visiting nurse, and one from the hospital, but he is unsure which one he should follow. He had not been weighing himself at home so had not noticed the weight gain, but called the ambulance because his ankles were swollen and he was having difficulty breathing.

- How would patient activation by entering daily weights into a tele-health application improve the outcomes for this patient?

- How might health information technology be tailored to the needs and preferences of this vulnerable patient?

Case 3. Home Care

A home care nurse visits a 68-year-old patient who was recently seen in a major academic medical center with a pressure ulcer. The nurse has a brief referral from the specialty practice requesting wound care and pain management, but no information related to the progression of the wound or how pain has been managed. When the home care nurse arrives, the patient is in bed and complaining of a pain. Upon assessment, the nurse finds that the patient has a pain level of 7/10 and is constipated. The pressure ulcer on the patient's sacrum is unstagable with green purulent drainage. The patient reports that her daughter is ill so she was unable to go to the pharmacy to pick up her prescriptions. Therefore, patient does not have any of the medications that were ordered for her. The patient reports that she was given a packet of papers as she was leaving the specialty clinic but that she left them in the ambulette and, therefore, does not have a copy of her medication list or her instructions.

- How would patient entry of actual medication use through interactive phone voice technology have triggered support for this family and patient adherence?

Case 4. Primary Care

A 47-year-old woman calls and makes an urgent care appointment. When she arrives, she tells the nurse practitioner that she has been having chest pain. The NP has never seen the patient before. From the electronic problem list it is clear that the patient has a history of CAD and sees a cardiologist in the community. However, there is no interoperability between the specialty clinic and primary care clinic. There are no stress test results, and no information about past reports of angina or how they were managed. On further questioning, the patient reports that she was told by her cardiologist to take nitroglycerin for chest pain. The NP at the primary care office places multiple phone calls to the cardiologist who is out of town and must decide whether to admit the patient to the hospital. There is incomplete information there as well, which is likely to lead to unnecessary duplicate testing.

- How would a clinical summary improve the NP's ability to effectively triage the patient and potentially avoid a hospital admission, given the severity of her complaint?
- How might this patient be involved in the development of the clinical summary?

Case 5. Long-Term Care (LTC)

An 88-year-old LTC patient and family complete an advanced directive (AD) with the LTC physician and the nurse director. The AD form is scanned and stored in the historical progress note section of the EMR. One week later, the patient develops a fever, cough, and new disorientation at 11 p.m. The nurse on duty looks for the AD but cannot find it in the EMR. A decision is made to send the deteriorating patient to the ED of a local hospital and the patient is transported without knowledge of an existing AD. The patient desaturates in the ambulance, is intubated in the ED, and then admitted to the intensive care unit (ICU). The family comes in the next morning and says that they want the patient sent back to the LTC facility with comfort measures only. The family is upset that patient was intubated as they took a day off from work to complete the advance directives form a week earlier to prevent this type of situation from occurring.

- How would a health information exchange ensure that the patient's goals of care are met?

Summary of Case Studies

In each of these cases, information was not available to the provider or patients and families at the right time leading to suboptimal care coordination. In each situation, health information technology could have enhanced patient engagement and improved the outcomes. As noted in Table 1, different types of HIT are useful and available to support a range of care coordination activities.

NURSING'S ROLE IN HIT ADOPTION

Clearly HIT is a critical mechanism to effective care coordination. However, it is important to have insight into the current status of HIT development and adoption. To that end, in 2012, the NQF contracted with Brigham and Women's Hospital in Boston to conduct both a literature review and site visits focused on the current HIT status designed to improve transfer of information during transitions of care, with a focus on quality measurement (Samal et al., 2012).

The main objective for this project was to assess the readiness of respondent organizations to transmit electronic data, to use HIT systems to perform the data capture, to standardize data, to communicate a patient-centered care plan, and use data for quality measurement. The results indicate that organizations are working to address care coordination demands, but are struggling with a patchwork of homegrown and commercial systems across settings, few of which connect and exchange data. Many organizations are still working to transfer basic discharge summaries electronically between settings, and organizations are using multiple methods for communicating and extracting the data that they need for care transitions. Where more comprehensive electronic methods do exist, they tend to be discipline-specific and focused on high-risk patients (Samal et al., 2012).

HIT in the broadest aspect has the potential to facilitate care coordination across all care settings. However, there are both technological and human factors that have slowed both the development and adoption of HIT. Technology factors related to matching devices to workflow, standards for interfacing infusion pumps and other medical devices with EHRs, user-interface design to support the task at hand as well as the role of the user (nurse, patient, consumer), and costs of technology all play a role in HIT adoption. This is further complicated by the inherent complexity of care coordination activities, which makes integration of HIT complex. Many of the existing EHRs fail to interoperate across different care delivery organizations. This is a huge barrier since as patients transition from acute to long-term and home care, the data from the EHR fails to move with the patient, putting the receiving care delivery team at risk when caring for patients. For this reason, many of the hand-offs that occur during care coordination are dependent on nurses to manually exchange, either through phone, fax, or hard copy documents, the information necessary for transferring responsibility of the patient.

Nurses play an important role in the development, implementation, and sustained adoption of HIT to support care coordination. This role is at the policy, care-delivery, and interprofessional levels. Nurses design, implement, and evaluate HIT projects to ensure all aspects of HIT support evidence-based, person-centered nursing practice. This involves leadership roles within organizations; providing input into the technical design by working with engineering experts; teaching nurses, patients, and consumers how to use HIT to support care coordination; providing testimony at the national level to guide future policies on HIT adoption; and conducting research to evaluate the impact of HIT on care outcomes.

Nurses also play a strong leadership role in vendor settings, pushing for the development of HIT that exemplifies nursing practice, while also showing the return on investment for such development. Through research nurses are participating in the development of new models for care coordination, using HIT as the foundation to bridge current care coordination gaps. The aforementioned areas are the responsibility of every practicing nurse, not just those formally involved in HIT or informatics roles.

FUTURE DIRECTIONS FOR HIT IN CARE COORDINATION

The development and integration of HIT within health care offers great promise. The explosion of mobile devices is providing a powerful tool for both patients and providers to track patient progress, share information, and communicate as patients move between office visits, the home, and inpatient settings. The increase in patient use and adoption of HIT is supplementing existing repositories of EHR data, thereby providing tremendous opportunities for data mining and healthcare analytics. Through this mining, nurses are able to identify which patients will benefit from care coordination and interventions that have the highest impact on outcomes.

HIT is no longer confined to care delivery settings as patients have mobile devices in their homes for tracking blood glucose and blood pressure and are even wearing these devices for continuous monitoring and transmission of the data to EHRs for real-time analysis. The future will bring a greater degree of connected devices allowing for robust data analytics. This is occurring in parallel with the advancement of data standards to support a nationally accepted structure for care plans, which is an important underpinning of care coordination. As these advances unfold, the role of nursing is essential as nurses bridge the space between the interprofessional team and patients and consumers across all domains of care.

HIT is evolving rapidly to advance care coordination through information exchange and decision support across multiple providers and settings. It can be expected to have a profound influence on the future of care coordination. As HIT is infused into care coordination processes, we will learn much about its role in supporting and facilitating this work. The data it provides will be a vital source of new knowledge to drive improvement and innovation. Nurses and other professionals engaged in care coordination can anticipate many important opportunities to shape future refinements of HIT and to champion its adoption and full integration into practice.

REFERENCES

Agency for Healthcare Research and Quality (AHRQ). (2011). Chapter 3. Care coordination measurement framework. In *Care coordination measures atlas elements of the framework.* Retrieved from http://www.ahrq.gov/professionals/systems/long-term-care/resources/coordination/atlas/chapter3.html

Alliance for Health Reform. (n.d.). A reporter's toolkit: Health information technology. Retrieved from http://www.allhealth.org/publications/health_information_technology/health_information_technology_toolkit.asp

Congressional Budget Office. (2008). Evidence on the costs and benefits of health information technology. Retrieved from http://www.cbo.gov/sites/default/files/cbofiles/ftpdocs/91xx/doc9168/05-20-healthit.pdf

Harle, C., Huerta, T., Ford, E., Diana, M., & Menachemi, N. (2013). Overcoming challenges to achieving meaningful use: Insights from hospitals that successfully received Centers for Medicare and Medicaid Services payments in 2011. *Jam Med Inform Assoc, 20,* 233–223.

Healthcare Information and Management Systems Society (HIMSS). (2003). HIMSS electronic health record definitional model: Version 1.0, 1–8. Retrieved from http://www.himss.org/ content/files/EHRAttributes.pdf

HealthIT.gov. (n.d.-a). Basics of health it. Retrieved from http://www.healthit.gov/patients-families/basics-health-it

HealthIT.gov. (n.d.-b). Answer to your question. Retrieved from http://www.healthit.gov/providers-professionals/faqs/what-patient-portal

Hersch, W. (2009). A stimulus to define informatics and health information technology. *BMC Medical Informatics and Decision Making, 9,* 24.

International Medical Informatics Association News (IMIA). (2009). IMIA-NI definition of nursing informatics updated. Retrieved from http://imianews.wordpress.com/2009/08/24/imia-ni-definition-of-nursing-informatics-updated/

Mell, P., & Grance, T. (2011). *The NIST definition of cloud computing, recommendations of the National Institute of Standards and Technology, U.S. Department of Commerce.* Washington, DC: Department of Commerce.

National Cancer Institute at the National Institutes of Health. (2012). *Evaluating online sources of health information.* Bethesda, MD: Author.

National Quality Forum (NQF). (2006). *National Quality Forum-endorsed definition and framework for measuring care coordination.* Washington, DC: Author.

National Quality Strategy (NQS). (2012). Retrieved from http://www.ahrq.gov/workingforquality/

Samal L., Dykes P. C., Greenberg J., Hasan O., Venkatesh A. K., Volk . A., & Bates, D. W. (2012). *Environmental analysis of health information technology to support care coordination and care transitions.* Washington, DC: National Quality Forum.

U.S. Government Printing Office. (2009) American Recovery and Reinvestment Act of 2009. Retrieved from http://frwebgate.access.gpo.gov/cgi-bin/getdoc.cgi?dbname=111_ cong_bills&docid=f:h1enr.pdf

Section 4

Transforming Healthcare Practice and Policy

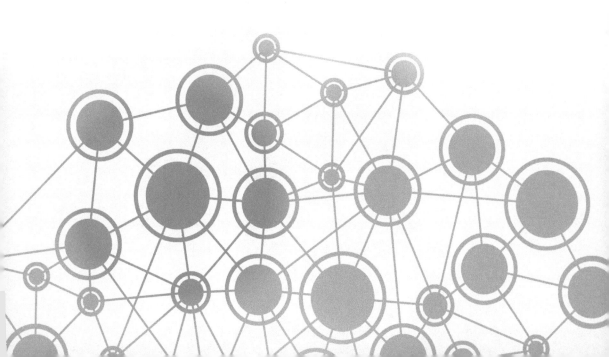

Chapter 10

Coordinating Care through Authentic Partnerships with Patients and Families

Richard Antonelli, MD, MS and Gina Rogers

ffective care coordination requires communication, collaboration, and a sense of accountability among the care team members. Several definitions of care coordination exist, and each of them emphasizes the central principles of communication, transparency, and cooperation (McDonald et al., 2010, 4–10; NQF, 2006; Antonelli, 2009). At the foundation of coordinating care across multiple providers is the notion of a coherent team which shares accountability across disciplines. There are many barriers to achieving effective coordination, including lack of time of the busy professionals involved, differences in workflow patterns preventing overlap in availability, difficulties associated with obtaining reimbursement for the time spent, confidentiality and privacy issues, barriers from entrenched professional hierarchies and institutional cultural biases, clinical specialties with different vocabularies and acronyms, and data transfer technology interface incompatibilities.

This chapter examines the ways various members of the care team may work together to support care coordination activities within the context of the specific elements and functions of the care coordination process, and offers tools and strategies to support improved interprofessional practice, enhanced communication, and information sharing. Using structured tools and methods must become a part of standard practice. In addition, proactive support from leadership, a changing policy environment, and workforce training that includes interprofessional education must also be promoted to achieve the collaboration among patients and their families and medical, social service, and educational providers necessary to minimize fragmentation in service delivery.

IDENTIFYING MEMBERS OF THE CARE TEAM

Central Role for Patients and Families

Delivery of care coordination services involves making connections among a set of service providers engaged in facilitating the delivery of appropriate health care and supporting services to meet an individual patient's needs. Every patient's healthcare team is unique: it has its own purpose, size, set of core members, operational settings, and methods of communication. The team engaged in coordinating care can be a simple triad: a primary care provider connecting the patient with a sub-specialist. However, for adults with multiple chronic conditions and children and youth with special healthcare needs (CYSHCNs), with their complex and often lifelong need for special services, truly integrated and broadly defined multidisciplinary teams must work together to coordinate care.

The challenges inherent in effectively coordinating care are dramatically illustrated in Figure 1, which is one parent's map of her child's care network (Lind, 2012). Coordinating in-home care and an extensive web of healthcare system participants, school services, and community resources can become a full-time job. In fact, data from a national survey shows that 24% of parents of children with special healthcare needs spend over five

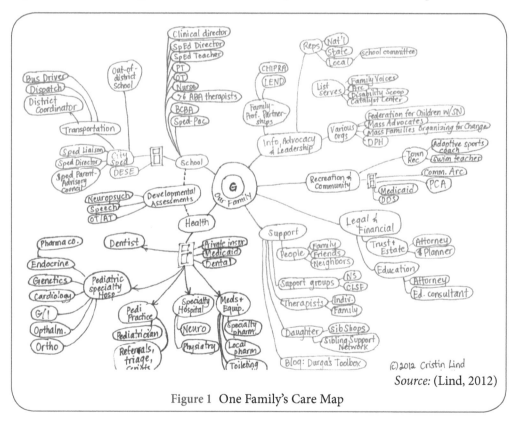

Source: (Lind, 2012)

Figure 1 One Family's Care Map

hours a week coordinating care, and over half of those spend more than 11 hours each week. These families clearly need help, with 42% reporting they are not getting the care coordination services they need (NS-CSHCNs, 2009–2010).

The patient/child and family's role at the center of the interconnections requires their active engagement in the care coordination process; they are often the only ones with connections to all the different components. However, important skill building is required for them to play that role, and for providers and care coordinators to support them. As Lind (2012, paragraph 5) notes, "The night I sketched out our complex web for the first time, I felt accomplished. I could see all the connections that I was managing. No wonder we had so many piles of unfolded laundry! I also felt called to action by how segmented and complicated the system was. It strengthened my commitment to be an agent for change."

The call for greater patient engagement goes beyond just this central role that connects all the different care team members. Studies overwhelmingly show the connection between patient and family engagement and improvements in physical and behavioral health, as well as reductions in costs (e.g., James, 2013; Hibbard and Green, 2013; Marcum, Sevick, & Handler, 2013). Their willingness and motivation to adhere to medication regimes, to tackle behavior changes like stopping smoking, and stick to behavioral health treatments all require their active participation in setting goals, in choosing wherever possible from qualified providers to deliver services, and in identifying other supports for planning and care coordination.

Working Effectively as a Team

Effective team-based collaboration in delivering care coordination services is fundamental to success. The underlying assumption is that optimal patient- and family-centered outcomes are the result of relationships in which patients and their families participate in a fully informed partnership with their primary care provider and a supportive, proactive healthcare team. Care coordination is the ingredient necessary to operationalize care processes leading to the achievement of these outcomes (Antonelli, 2009). Achieving the desired outcomes then requires attention to the key drivers of effective teamwork. The set of principles in Table 1 summarizes these key drivers, distilled by the Institute of Medicine Best Practices Innovation Collaborative from evidence from seminal works such as Wagner's (2001) Chronic Care Model and Bodenheimer's (2007) experiences building teams in primary care.

Table 1 Principles of Team-Based Health Care

Shared goals: The team—including the patient and, where appropriate, family members or other support persons—works to establish shared goals that reflect patient and family priorities, and can be clearly articulated, understood, and supported by all team members.
Clear roles: There are clear expectations for each team member's functions, responsibilities, and accountabilities, which optimize the team's efficiency and often make it possible for the team to take advantage of division of labor, thereby accomplishing more than the sum of its parts.
Mutual trust: Team members earn each other's trust, creating strong norms of reciprocity and greater opportunities for shared achievement.
Effective communication: The team prioritizes and continuously refines its communication skills. It has consistent channels for candid and complete communication, which are accessed and used by all team members across all settings.
Measurable processes and outcomes: The team agrees on and implements reliable and timely feedback on successes and failures in both the functioning of the team and achievement of the team's goals. These are used to track and improve performance immediately and over time.

Source: Mitchell et al., 2012

One fundamental starting point for the care coordination team is to clearly identify the roles and responsibilities for each team member. However, because of the wide variety of circumstances under which care coordination will be employed, the delivery of care coordination services needs to be flexible and vary by location, encounter type, timing, intensity, and duration. Care providers must take into account the cultural preferences of each family and strive for effectiveness in different circumstances and environments. Innovative approaches to care are essential, from face-to-face visits to nontraditional encounters that optimize the use of resources and maximize value for families and providers (Antonelli, 2009).

Similarly, assessing the set of care coordination *functions* that need to be performed and then matching tasks based on expertise and availability across the full array of team members will be more effective than creating prescriptive rules around education levels and credentialing under a formal "care coordinator" role. Care coordination is comprised of a set of activities (Antonelli, 2009) and is often implemented by a variety of personnel, including the patients themselves, their families, their caregivers, nurses, nurse practitioners, physicians, medical assistants, social workers, nursing assistants, pharmacists, community health workers, case managers, and patient advocates. As a result, these various coordinators may come from the patient's own home or from a variety of community-based entities. In partnership with activated patients and families, the various members of the care team must coalesce around a specific set of care goals, captured in the patient-centered and patient-driven care plan.

While an individual may be designated as a care coordinator, it is essential to understand that the specific responsibilities for that role should be identified on a patient/family-specific basis. At times, the patient and family serve exclusively as their own care coordinator. However, the attribution of this role to the patient/family/caregiver should always be an active process performed in conjunction with the needs and preferences of the patient and family.

The care team must include an accountable person who is ultimately responsible for assuring that the patient and family are fully engaged in the process, and that each team member is able to deliver upon their respective care goals.

One framework for defining the key domains of care coordination services is provided in Table 2. Strategies for identifying roles and responsibilities for each of these domains are described in the next section, including case studies that illustrate their application.

Table 2 Key Domains and Activities of Patient-Centered and Team-Based Care Coordination

Needs assessment for care coordination and continuing care coordination engagement
- Family-driven, youth-guided needs assessment, goal setting
- Use a standard process to assess care coordination needs (differs from clinical needs)
- Engage team, assign clear roles and responsibilities
- Develop authentic family–provider/care team partnerships; requires family/youth capacity building, professional skill building

Care planning and communication
- Family and care team co-develop care plans
- Ensure communication among all members of the care team
- Monitor, follow-up, respond to change, track progress toward goals
- Workforce training occurs that promotes effective care plan implementation

Facilitating care transitions (inpatient, ambulatory)
- Family engagement to align transition plan with family goals, needs
- Implement components of successful transitions (eight elements, including receiving provider and acknowledging responsibility)
- Ensure information needed at transition points is available

Connecting with community resources and schools
- Facilitate connection to family-run organization/family partner
- Coordinate services with schools, agencies, payers
- Identify opportunities to reduce duplication of efforts in building knowledge of available community services

Transitioning to adult care (for children), self-care skill development
- Implement Center for Health Care Transition Improvement's Six Core Elements of Health Care Transition (HCT)
- Teach/model self-care skills, communication skills, self-advocacy

Source: Massachusetts Child Health Quality Coalition Care Coordination Task Force, funded by the Centers for Medicare and Medicaid Services (CMS) through grant funds issued pursuant to CHIPRA section 401(d) (Care Coordination Task Force, Rogers, Antonelli, & Leadholm, 2013)

A FRAMEWORK FOR CARE COORDINATION

The five domains in this framework are generalizable across all ages. It is critically important to note that *this framework is relevant to support the provision of care coordination, irrespective of the type of care need being addressed*. For example, whether a patient is an 80-year old person being referred to a specialized nursing facility following an acute cardiovascular event, or whether we are focusing on referring a newborn for a home visiting program following an uneventful delivery, the activities of care coordination are uniform. This framework offers a process by which roles and responsibilities for each care team member can be specified.

Domain 1. Needs Assessment for Care Coordination, Continuing Engagement

The first step in the care coordination process is needs assessment and goal setting. Working with individuals and families to identify their care coordination needs and preferences, and then providing the individuals with the opportunity to choose care that fits with their personal preferences, such as the setting, time of day, and where to receive care, increases patient engagement and enhances the likelihood that care will align with their goals and enhance their quality of life.

There remains much work to be done to effectively develop authentic family–provider partnerships. An Institute of Medicine workshop on partnering with patients (IOM, 2013) offered some key messages on creating central roles for patients. Being an engaged patient requires skill development; not everyone comes to the table with a comfort level and willingness to ask questions. Similarly, actively engaging patients is not intuitive for providers either. Patients and clinicians learn these skills over time and through partnership with a supportive care team. Important culture change must come first. Providers must learn how to listen and listen fully.

The team-based planning process of the National Wraparound Initiative, designed for children with complex emotional, behavioral, or mental health difficulties, offers tools for achieving family-driven goal setting, with demonstrated success in better outcomes. Improved outcomes are attributed to better treatment acceptability and family/child engagement, agreement about treatment goals, increased self-efficacy, and better use of social supports including other families with lived experience (National Wraparound Initiative, 2011). Table 3 provides an overview of a structured process of an initial meeting to assess strengths, needs, and setting goals with the family.

Table 3 Typical Process for an Initial Care Planning Meeting: Wraparound Services for Children with Serious Emotional Disturbance

- Introducing the team, reviewing progress
- Ground rules
- Share the family's vision
- Team develops its mission
- What are the "Big Worries"?
- What are the two or three needs and goals that we will start with?
  - Select a goal and determine the first few objectives (first steps)
  - What will be the measurement strategy to know if the plan is working?
  - Strengths and culture are reviewed, expanded, and discussed
  - Options are "brainstormed" to achieve the objective
  - Specific tasks or action steps are agreed upon and assigned
  - Tasks are written concretely—who will specifically do what by when
- What is the implementation plan? When will the team meet again? How will communication take place between meetings?
- Who are we missing? Do we have everyone we need to implement this plan? Who do we need at future meetings to continue planning?
- Risk management/safety planning review (if needed)
- Consent forms: permission to provide services, for facilitator to speak with other team members
- Follow up meeting is scheduled (if necessary)

Source: Irsfeld, 2013

Domain 2. Care Planning and Communication

The needs assessment and goal setting processes lead to the next set of care coordination activities: the co-development of a care plan. The steps include ensuring communication among all members of the care team, discussing roles and responsibilities and writing them into the care plan, and identifying ways to monitor, follow-up, respond to change, and track progress toward goals as expressed in the care plan. Successful care coordination based on the goals contained within a single, dynamic care plan is an essential tool for optimal, multidisciplinary care coordination. This centrally accessible care plan will be implemented in various fashions, depending upon local assets and capabilities. For example:

- Is the care plan linked to the electronic health record (EHR)?
- Does the patient have access to it in a personal health record or patient portal?
- Can it be provided in non-electronic format?
- Can other disciplines such as pharmacy provide input to the care plan?
- Do those outside the system initiating the care plan have access?

- Are there procedures in place to explain confidentiality issues and then for the patient/family to provide consents as needed for the sharing of information?

- Recognize that, where EHR systems are not in place, the patient is often called upon to serve as the conduit for ensuring all members of the care team have access to information in the care plan.

The care plan supports team-based care by providing a vehicle for ensuring that all members of the care team are on the same page. The case study of a child receiving services from multiple state agencies (see Case Study 1) provides an example of the different accountabilities involved in a case where community supports, as well as medical and psychiatric services, are elements of the care plan.

Case Study 1: Child Receiving Services from Multiple Providers and Agencies

Lizbeth is a seven–year-old girl and the second child. She was diagnosed with cerebral palsy when she was six months old and began receiving early intervention (EI) services under the state's Department of Public Health services when she was a year old. She demonstrated delays in gross and fine motor skills and the EI services were helpful in teaching Lizbeth and her parents how to stretch her legs and arms, strengthen her physical capabilities, and improve her motor skills. Although Lizbeth had always been small for her age, she was a happy child and her parents and older brother doted on her. As Lizbeth got older, she expressed frustration in her physical limitations and her inability to play with other children and her older brother like other children without limitations. She was mainstreamed in her local school and seemed to enjoy going off to the same school her brother attended. The school nurse was a key advocate who supported her inclusion in the classroom.

Over six months, Lizbeth began to withdraw, express frustration with school, and refused to do her school work and her physical exercises. She had difficulty sleeping through the night and had to be cajoled into eating. It wasn't clear what precipitated the decline and whether neurological changes were occurring. Her parents noted mood swings and that she wasn't that happy little girl anymore. They brought Lizbeth to her primary care provider for an evaluation. The nurse practitioner performed a comprehensive examination, including a standard neurologic assessment. The results were inconclusive. The nurse practitioner contacted a child and adolescent psychiatrist available through a state psychiatry referral program (the Massachusetts Child Psychiatry Access Project (MCPAP) and consulted with the MD. Both providers agreed it made sense to complete additional tests, and the psychiatrist agreed to see Lizbeth. The social worker's intake included asking if the family had ever looked into any of the community-based resources for families of children with cerebral palsy or the Children's Behavioral Health Initiative (CBHI) under the state's Medicaid program. The family was pleased to hear about these resources but expressed their desire to have some support in navigating what might be a series of referrals across multiple organizations and agencies. After all, these inter-connections were new to them, and their experience in the past indicated that it can be challenging for families to find the most efficient path without guidance.

Members of the care team engaged in coordinating care

The family, school, teacher, school nurse, pediatric primary care provider (nurse practitioner), psychiatrist, social worker, community supports, and Lizbeth's expanding social network.

Actions

- The mother agreed to contact the Department of Mental Health's (DMH) family resource center and was connected to a family support group through the local chapter.
- Social worker, serving in role as care coordinator, met with the mother and Lizbeth and assessed her broad needs. Made referral to community-based resources.
- Child psychiatrist provided a more thorough evaluation and did not feel medication was indicated at this point.
- DMH Children's Services staff talked to the mother and helped her get a referral to the local Community Service agency.
- Provider completed evaluation and family agreed that Intensive Care Coordination services were indicated as many issues needed further exploration.
- Primary care provider received recommendations from the social worker and the psychiatrist. She reviewed these with the patient and family. A care plan was created which reflected all the care needs for Lizbeth.
- The family was pleased that Lizbeth was re-integrated into the school, and the school nurse was a key advocate on her behalf.

Source: Case study provided by Barbara Leadholm, Principal, Health Management Associates, and former Commissioner MA Department of Mental Health and Senior Advisor, MassHealth Office of Behavioral Health.

There is a wide range of functionality and detail provided in care plans, and there are definite trade-offs in time spent developing and then maintaining the accuracy of the information they contain. Different formats and level of detail are required in different circumstances. The necessary detail for sharing the clinical information needed for effective decision-making and reducing duplication of tests and treatments can make them less useful as references for patients and families. Many programs have developed a variety of patient-focused materials, such as asthma action plans, to provide more easily understandable guidance for daily and emergency care, showing what to do when different symptoms occur, identifying triggers, and understanding how to control things that make the condition worse.

Domain 3. Facilitating Care Transitions (Inpatient, Ambulatory)

A range of care coordination functions is required to facilitate transitions at discharge from inpatient settings and when referrals are made to other providers and caregivers. Strategies for using care coordination to reduce readmissions following transitions from inpatient stays have already been provided in Chapter 7, and these highlight the critical importance of each member of the patient-centered care team.

These approaches can be expanded to apply to referrals more broadly, including transitions from primary care to subspecialty providers and nursing providers to community-based support agencies. These transitions occur across personnel, agencies, and settings. The following key ingredients are required to ensure a successful transition:

- Aligns with family goals and respects the patient's view about the handoff
- Timely
- Well-informed
- Transparent to the patient/family
- Family is supported to initiate the referral request when appropriate
- Receiving provider acknowledges responsibility
- New team composition, goals, and tasks are articulated into care management plan
- Backed by a system that can track that it occurred

The case of Juanita, an adolescent whose chronic illness has resulted in multiple unplanned inpatient readmissions, illustrates the opportunity for team-based care that addresses and tracks medical, social, and emotional needs across the community continuum (see Case Study 2). Numerous providers and settings play an important role in helping Juanita and her family implement a plan that will enable Juanita to feel better

Case Study 2: Chronically Ill Youth with Multiple Unplanned Inpatient Readmissions

Juanita is a 16-year-old female who has a history of moderate, persistent asthma. She lives with her mother and brother in an urban setting in an apartment building that was built 60 years ago. The apartment has forced hot air heat that does not always work well and is plagued by rodent infestation. Although there is no smoking in her apartment, there are multiple cigarette smokers on her floor in the building. The road in front of her apartment is used frequently by trucks, often idling for hours while they await unloading at a distribution center located on her block.

It has been a challenging year in school for Juanita, having missed about 45 days due to two hospital admissions for asthma in the last five months. She has also missed school on days when she stayed home because she felt that her breathing would not allow her to make it through the school day. The school is concerned that Juanita may not be able to pass to the next grade at the end of the current academic year. This has Juanita and her family quite sad.

Juanita has a primary care provider in her community, but she needs to take three different buses to get there. She has seen a pulmonologist in the past, but that was during an inpatient stay. These providers have prescribed a regimen of three different medications that she is supposed to take every day.

Her insurance coverage has been problematic, since her family's eligibility for coverage lapses every year. She is eventually able to be reinstated for insurance coverage, but it does lead to her having gaps in obtaining the necessary maintenance and "rescue" medications to keep her asthma in check.

Implications

This case study demonstrates the need for effective care coordination across the following multiple settings and the interventions in each setting in order to reduce the risk of rehospitalizations.

1. Family's Home
   a. *Interventions*: Environmental assessment, risk abatement, patient and family education
2. School
   a. *Interventions:* School nurse aware and proactively checks in with Juanita

(continued)

Case Study 2 (continued)

    b. Asthma action plan available

    c. School nurse has permission to contact primary care and specialist providers

    d. Teachers and school administration link with medical team to flag issues of attendance and academic achievement (with family's permission)

3. Health and Chronic Illness Care

    a. *Interventions:* Primary care tracks asthma control both by office visits and proactive outreach, especially following inpatient stays and Emergency Department stays for asthma

    b. Primary care provider assesses how Juanita is adapting to the stresses of her poorly controlled asthma, including her feelings about possibly not graduating this year

    c. Pulmonologist works with patient and family, as well as with PCP, to define optimal means for Juanita to access services when she is not feeling well

    d. Inpatient team works with Juanita and her family, prior to discharge, to understand what triggered need for admission:

        i.   Failure of her current treatment regimen

        ii. Lack of access to medications

        iii. Environmental issues (e.g., rodents, dust, cigarette exposure, etc.)

4. Community Resources

    a. *Interventions:* Referrals to community agencies to assess housing, transportation, insurance coverage

    b. Outreach to community health advocates to address issue of mitigation of environmental risk of prolonged diesel exhaust exposure

Source: Case study provided by Richard C. Antonelli, MD, Boston Children's Hospital.

and learn to manage her asthma effectively at home and at school. Transition planning includes communication about how the care plan will be managed by Juanita, her family, and members of her care team. Each individual needs to know essential information, such as where the plan will be located, how to access it, how often it will evaluated and updated, by whom, and who is responsible for making sure that members of the care team are alerted to any changes.

Domain 4. Connecting to Community Resources

Care coordination functions as seen from the primary care perspective, especially within the context of a medical home, require developing and sustaining relationships with community providers and agencies. Examples run the gamut from state and local agency programs within departments of mental and public health, foster care, and the criminal justice systems to visiting nurse associations, tobacco quit lines, nutrition counseling and exercise programs, and alcohol and drug counseling. In interviews with families, a high priority is put on linking to family-run organizations, and connecting to someone else who has already been through the experience who can help navigate the connections that will have to be made and identify education needs. More systems are developing paid roles for family partners, patient navigators, and community health workers, all of whom bring cultural sensitivity to delivering important care coordination services. Physicians, nurses, and other members of the care team from the medical and behavioral health communities need to learn how to work with these resources more effectively.

The two case studies presented above both contain important community connections with identified roles for different members of the care team. Building trust among these different participants requires an understanding of different work flows and responsibilities. Often, health information systems cannot communicate easily between the medical and the community settings. A promising wave of new technologies, however, are offering capacity that includes adequate security for medical and sensitive behavioral health issues that can be used to facilitate "virtual huddles" with social service resources and community mental health facilities.

Domain 5. Transitioning to Adult Care, Self-Care Skill Development

Supporting the transition from pediatric to adult care is a special care coordination domain that applies to adolescent and young adult populations. The Center for Health Care Transition Improvement (CHCTI) has developed a set of tools to support care coordination activities between these two very different systems (CHCTI/Got Transitions, n.d.). They developed a six-item Health Care Transition Index identifying the following steps to a successful transition: creation of a specific health policy governing transition; identification of transitioning youth whose progress is tracked in a registry; development of knowledge and skills for all members of the care team to support transition; a specific process by which the youth is prepared for transition; working with the youth and family to plan for a successful transition; and enabling the actual transfer of care once the youth is ready.

Teaching and modeling self-care skills, communication skills, and self-advocacy are important components of the transition process that also apply to care coordination needs in other situations. The importance of identifying who within the care team is best suited to undertake these activities was noted by Bodenheimer (2007) in his conversations with California physicians. Many of them worry about who has sufficient skills to undertake self-management support functions, since physicians are shouldering too much of the responsibility, an unsustainable strategy as the burden of chronic illness continues to increase.

CARE COORDINATION FUNCTIONS LINKED TO OUTCOMES

Care coordination has been cited by the Institute of Medicine (2001) as a cross-cutting element to close the "quality chasm". Why has it been so challenging to implement successful care coordination programs? There are at least two explanations.

First, there has been a systematic lack of interdisciplinary performance to support care coordination across all components of the health delivery system. These functions have often been focused on inpatient management. Or, they have been provided through the auspices of case managers, often housed within insurers.

The second reason for this lack of systemic, interdisciplinary care coordination performance is reflected in this adage: "If you can't measure something, you can't improve it. And you can't measure something until you define it!" One of the first measures of care coordination, the Care Coordination Measurement Tool (CCMT), assesses care coordination activities, the time commitment to perform those activities, and the outcomes of those activities (Antonelli, Stille, & Antonelli, 2008). The elements of this practical data collection tool for defining the activities of care coordination and identifying performance of those activities by members of the care team are provided in Table 4 (see page 182). Early work with the CCMT has suggested its utility in documenting improved quality and financial outcomes in patients with specific care needs, such as children with asthma in community-based, pediatric primary care practices. For sustainable care coordination funding, proof statements from projects that track the time spent on care coordination and then relate that to system cost savings and quality and safety metrics, with links to patient experience, must be put into wider use.

CAPACITY BUILDING: WORKFORCE TRAINING, AND INTERPROFESSIONAL EDUCATION

How do we build capacity in care coordination to meet current and future demands? We must begin with a new paradigm for training: effective care coordination will only result from multidisciplinary, interprofessional learning opportunities. These shared learning teams must include participants from nursing, social work, behavioral health, medicine, community service providers, case management, and care coordination. Patients, families, and caregivers must play a central role, as both teachers and co-learners. Preparation for effective care coordination requires a strong foundation in teamwork and collaboration. Team members need to be confident in their ability to describe each person's role and accountabilities, to communicate important information, and to activate team and community resources (IPEC, 2012). The recent growth in interprofessional education in the United States is making teamwork training more accessible for all professionals. Many of these programs may be customized for local insights, experiences, and needs (Antonelli, Browning, Hackett-Hunter, McAllister, & Risko, 2012).

Education on techniques for improving communication and teamwork must be an important component of this capacity building. Many such techniques have been integrated successfully into activities supporting culture change to promote patient safety, including multidisciplinary rounding, short team "huddles," and structured communication forms such as the Situation Background Assessment Recommendation (SBAR). Building care coordination "rounds," where direct care coordination efforts are discussed and the input of all colleagues can be heard, support having conversations where challenging issues can be discussed with all care team members. Also, tools like the SBAR form offer teams a solution to bridge the gap in communication, including hand-offs, patient transfers, critical conversations, and telephone calls. It creates a shared expectation between the sender and receiver of the information being shared.

Work identifying core competencies for interprofessional collaborative practice (Interprofessional Education Collaborative, 2011; Pediatrics Milestone Working Group, 2012) has established specific competencies for interprofessional communication, teams, and team work and offers learning activities and examples. Real culture change, where authentic patient/family-provider relationships guide care coordination decisions, will require coupling the workforce training with accountability systems for assessing organizational supports that guarantee effective, patient-centered communication with people from diverse populations. This is necessary for ensuring that leadership commitment, workforce development, language services, and health literacy are all brought to bear on the care coordination work. That is the challenge and the promise from building working relationships among the family/youth, clinicians, community partners, and other professionals to support care coordination that delivers on all three components of the Triple Aim: improvement of health, improvement in the patient experience, and decreasing cost of care (Berwick, Nolan, & Whittington, 2008).

Table 4 Care Coordination Functions and Outcomes in the Medical
Home Care Coordination Measurement Tool (CCMT)

Care Coordination Needs (choose all that apply)	Activity to Fulfill Needs (choose all that apply)
1. Make appointments	1. Telephone discussion with:
2. Follow-up referrals	a. Patient
3. Order prescriptions, supplies, services, etc.	b. Parent/family
4. Reconcile discrepancies	c. School
5. Coordination services (schools, agencies, payers, etc.)	d. Agency
	e. Hospital/clinic
Time Spent	f. Payer
1. less than 5 minutes	g. Voc/training
2. 5–9 minutes	h. Pharmacy
3. 10–19 minutes	2. Electronic (E-Mail) Contact with:
4. 20–29 minutes	a. Patient
5. 30–39 minutes	b. Parent
6. 40–49 minutes	c. School
7. 50 minutes and greater*	d. Agency
(*Please NOTE actual minutes if greater than 50)	e. Hospital/clinic
	f. Payer
	g. Voc./training
	h. Pharmacy
	3. Contact with Consultant
Staff	a. Telephone
RN, LPN, MD, NP, PA, MA, SW, Cler	b. Meeting
	c. Letter
Clinical Competence	d. E-Mail
C= Clinical competence required	4. Form Processing: (e.g., school, camp, or complex record release)
NC= Clinical competence not required	5. Confer with Primary Care Physician
	6. Written Report to Agency: (e.g., SSI)
	7. Written Communication
	a. E-Mail
	b. Letter
	8. Chart Review
	9. Patient-Focused Research
	10. Contact with Home Care Personnel
	a. Telephone
	b. Meeting
	c. Letter
	d. E-Mail
	11. Develop/Modify Written Care Plan
	12. Meeting/Case Conference

Outcome(s)	Outcome(s)
As a result of this care coordination activity, the following was PREVENTED (choose ONLY ONE, if applicable):	As a result of this care coordination activity, the following OCCURRED (choose all that apply):
1a. ER visit	2a. Advised family/patient on home management
1b. Subspecialist visit	2b. Referral to ER
1c. Hospitalization	2c. Referral to subspecialist
1d. Visit to pediatric office/clinic	2d. Referral for hospitalization
1e. Lab/X-ray	2e. Referral for pediatric sick office visit
1f. Specialized therapies (PT, OT, etc.)	2f. Referral to lab/X-ray
	2g. Referral to community agency
	2h. Referral to specialized therapies
	2i. Ordered prescription, equipment, diapers, taxi, etc.
	2j. Reconciled discrepancies (including missing data, miscommunications, compliance issues)
	2k. Reviewed labs, specialist reports, IEPs, etc.
	2l. Advocacy for family/patient
	2m. Met family's immediate needs, questions, concerns
	2n. Unmet needs (PLEASE SPECIFY)
	2o. Not applicable/Don't know
	2p. Outcome pending

Source: Antonelli, 2013

CONCLUSION

There may be no set of activities that are more dependent on high performing, interprofessional training and performance than care coordination. Fortunately, the evolution of health delivery systems will require implementation of interprofessional, team-based, patient- and family-centric care coordination. Employing frameworks which articulate roles, responsibilities, measures, and expected outcomes of this interprofessional effort will be essential.

REFERENCES

Antonelli, R. C. (2013). *Medical home care coordination measurement tool.* Boston, MA: Boston Children's Hospital.

Antonelli, R. C., Browning, D. M., Hackett-Hunter, P., McAllister, J. W., & Risko, W. (2012). Pediatric care coordination curriculum users' guide. Boston, MA: Boston Children's Hospital, funded through the Maternal and Child Health Bureau.

Antonelli, R. C., McAllister, J. W., & Popp, J. (2009). Making care coordination a critical component of the pediatric health system: A multidisciplinary framework. Volume 110 (May 21) The Commonwealth Fund. Retrieved http://www.commonwealth-fund.org/Publications/Fund-Reports/2009/May/Making-Care-Coordination-a-Critical-Component-of-the-Pediatric-Health-System.aspx

Antonelli, R. C., Stille, C. J., & Antonelli, D. M. (2008). Care coordination for children and youth with special health care needs: A descriptive, multisite study of activities, personnel costs, and outcomes. *Pediatrics, 122*, e209–e216.

Berry, J. G., Ziniel, S. I., Freeman, L., Kaplan, W., Antonelli, R. C., Gay, J., ... Goldmann, D. (2013). Hospital readmission and parent perceptions of their child's hospital discharge. *International Journal for Quality in Health Care*, 1–9.

Berwick, D. M., Nolan, T. W., & Whittington, J. (2008). The triple aim: Care, health, and cost. *Health Affairs, 27*(3), 759–69.

Bodenheimer, T. (2007). *Building teams in primary care: Lessons learned*. California HealthCare Foundation.

Care Coordination Task Force, Rogers G., Antonelli R. C., & Leadholm, B. (2013). Key elements of high-performing pediatric care coordination: Framework and mea-sures to monitor adoption. Massachusetts Child Health Quality Coalition (CHQC), funded by the Centers for Medicare and Medicaid Services (CMS) through grant funds issued pursuant to CHIPRA section 401(d), Quality Demonstration Grant.

Center for Health Care Transition Improvement/Got Transitions! (n.d.) Health Care Transition (HCT) Index. Retrieved from www.gottransition.org/6-core-elements

Hibbard, J. H., & Greene, J. (2013). What the evidence shows about patient activation: Better health outcomes and care experiences; fewer data on costs. *Health Affairs, 32*, 207–214.

Institute of Medicine (IOM) Planning Committee. (2013). Partnering with patients to drive shared decisions, better value, and care improvement. National Academy of the Sciences. Proceedings retrieved from www.iom.edu/partneringwithpatients

Institute of Medicine (IOM) Committee on Quality of Health Care in America. (2001). Crossing the quality chasm: A new health system for the 21st century. Washington, DC: National Academy Press.

Interprofessional Education Collaborative (IPEC). (2011). Core competencies for inter-professional collaborative practice. Retrieved from www.aacn.nche.edu/education-resources/ipecreport.pdf

Irsfeld, J. A. (2013). Unpublished training materials used by Community Healthlink Community Service Agency drawn from National Wraparound Initiative resources.

James, J. (2013). Health policy brief: Patient engagement. *Health Affairs*, 1–6. Retrieved from http://healthaffairs.org/healthpolicybriefs/brief_pdfs/healthpolicybrief_86.pdf

Lind, C. (2012). My care map, or the picture that tells a thousand words. Retrieved from http://durgastoolbox.com/2012/ 09/19/durga-tool-9-my-care-map-or-the-picture-that- tells-a-thousand-words/

Marcum, Z. A., Sevick, M. A., Handler, S. M. (2013). Medication nonadherence: A diagnosable and treatable medical condition. *Journal of the American Medical Association*, *309*(20), 2105–2106.

McAllister, J. W., Cooley, W. C., Van Cleave, J., Boudreau, A. A., & Kuhlthau, K. (2013). Medical home transformation in pediatric primary care—What drives change? *Annals of Family Medicine*, *11*(Suppl 1), S90–S98.

McAllister, J. W., Presler, E., & Cooley, W. C. (2007). *Medical home practice-based care coordination: A workbook*. Center for Medical Home Improvement (CMHI).

McDonald, K. M., Schultz, E., Albin, L., Pineda, N., Lonhart, J., Sundaram, V., … Malcolm, E. (2010). *Care coordination atlas version 3*. Rockville, MD: Agency for Healthcare Research and Quality (AHRQ).

Mitchell, P., Wynia, M., Golden, R., McNellis, B., Okun, S., Webb, C. E., Rohrbach, V., Van Kohorn, I. (2012). Core principles and values of effective team-based health care. Institute of Medicine (IOM). Retrieved from www.nationalahec.org/pdfs/VSRT-Team-Based-Care-Principles-Values.pdf

National Quality Forum (NQF). (2006). NQF-endorsed definition and framework for measuring and reporting care coordination. NQF, 1. Retrieved from http://www.ahrq.gov/professionals/systems/long-term-care/resources/coordination/atlas/care-coordination-measures-atlas.pdf

National Survey of Children with Special Health Care Needs. (NS-CSHCN).(2009–2010). Data query from the Child and Adolescent Health Measurement Initiative. Data Resource Center for Child and Adolescent Health. Retrieved from www.child-healthdata.org

National Wraparound Initiative. (2011). Resource guide to wraparound. Retrieved from www.nwi.pdx.edu/NWI-book/index.shtml

Pediatrics Milestone Working Group (2012). The pediatrics milestone project. The Accreditation Council for Graduate Medical Education (ACGME) and the American Board of Pediatrics (ABP). Retrieved from https://www.abp.org/abpwebsite/publicat/milestones.pdf

Wagner, E. H., Austin, B. T., Davis, C., Hindmarsh, M., Schaefer, J., Bonomi, A. (2001). Improving chronic illness care: Translating evidence into action. *Health Affairs*, *20*(6):64–78.

Chapter 11

Community-Based Care Transitions: From Care Coordination Pilot to CMS Program

Donna Zazworsky, MS, RN, CCM, FAAN

Health care is undergoing a transformation that is moving nursing into the forefront of change. No longer is quantity (the number of billable visits that a patient has with a provider, for example) the measure of success in health care. Today, one of the central goals in health care is to demonstrate value through improved quality and reduced costs. In order to achieve value, health systems are focused on efforts to make sure that the patient receives the right care at the right time from the right health professional or community resource. At the heart of this work is care coordination. This is where nursing plays a pivotal role in both the hospital and community settings.

The Affordable Care Act of 2010 introduced many new initiatives to improve health care and lower costs. One initiative, Hospital-Value-Based Purchasing (VBP), was designed to create incentives for hospitals to improve their performance on selected quality and safety measures. Under the VBP Program, hospitals will receive incentive payments for Medicare patients based on how well they perform on quality measures and how much they improve on each measure compared to a baseline period (CMS factsheet, 2013).

One visible example of VBP is hospital readmissions for specific diseases, such as heart failure, acute myocardial infarction, and community-acquired pneumonia. Hospitals that improve their readmission rates will receive an incentive for improved readmissions; hospitals that do not improve their rates will be penalized. Not surprisingly, most hospitals and healthcare systems around the United States are seeking strategies and programs to position themselves for success in VBP. The purpose of this chapter is to describe how one organization, the Carondelet Health Network in southern Arizona, seized the opportunity to improve care, reduce costs, and prepare for value-based purchasing through the development and testing of a nurse-led care coordination model to reduce hospital readmissions.

BUILDING ON A LONG HISTORY OF INNOVATIVE NURSE CARE COORDINATION

Carondelet Health Network (CHN) is the largest faith-based integrated health care system in southern Arizona. It is a member of Ascension Health, the largest Catholic health system in the United States. CHN has three hospitals: Carondelet St. Mary's Hospital (recognized as Arizona's first hospital) and Carondelet St. Joseph's Hospital, both located in Tucson, and Carondelet Holy Cross, a small, critical access hospital located along the Mexican–American border in Nogales, Arizona. Carondelet Medical Group, the primary care arm of the network, is a large group practice with more than 80 primary care physicians, nurse practitioners, and physician assistants. CHN also has Carondelet Specialty Group, a specialty practice comprised of cardiologists and cardiac/vascular surgeons.

Carondelet has a long history of innovation in nurse care coordination and community-based nursing practice (Lamb and Zazworsky, 2005). In the late 1980s, the nursing leadership at Carondelet St. Mary's Hospital initiated one of the first programs in which hospital-based nurses continued to care for their patients during their transition from hospital to home. The well-known "Carondelet Model" set the stage for today's transitional care and high-risk nurse case management programs.

In the late 1990s and early 2000, Carondelet was one of four Community Nursing Organizations (CNOs) in the country to test a capitated nurse case management model for Medicare beneficiaries. Each of the CNOs received a single payment for each person for nurse case management, home care, and medical equipment. Utilizing nurse partners for low- and moderate-risk patients and nurse case managers for high-risk patients, this program managed the outpatient care for over 2,000 Medicare members. This model resulted in improved health status, quality of life, and satisfaction for its members, but did not significantly reduce overall health costs for members compared to a randomized control group. Many of the lessons from the CNOs were incorporated in subsequent federal demonstrations on care coordination and case management.

Following the CNO demonstration, payment for care in most health systems shifted from capitated payment (where there is a preset amount of reimbursement for designated services) back to fee-for-service and for hospitals, back to payment based on diagnosis-related groupings (DRGs). Along with payment changes, the emphasis of care changed from managing the whole sequence of healthcare, back to a more silo-based or setting specific approach in which each setting focused on maximizing their own income. Carondelet's case management efforts shifted to more of an inpatient focus with the aim of managing hospital length of stay. Like most hospitals, this system worked well for Carondelet until CMS began introducing new initiatives around value-based purchasing.

Lessons from Carondelet's legacy in care coordination and case management were used to build the framework for Carondelet's programs to respond to penalties for hospital readmission rates and to prepare for the value-based purchasing program. Many of the interventions and tools developed and refined at Carondelet over previous decades, particularly nurse case management for high-risk patients, standardized risk assessment, and patient education instruments, were seen as essential to success in achieving targeted quality and cost-related goals.

REDISCOVERING CARE COORDINATION FOR A NEW TIME: THE HEART FAILURE TRANSITIONS PILOT

In the fall of 2010, Carondelet embarked on a series of strategic activities designed to improve the integration of services for high-risk populations, to reduce hospital readmissions, and to improve quality outcomes. One goal was to reduce 30-day hospital readmissions for individuals admitted with heart failure. At the time, the readmission rate for this population was well over the national norm and was expected to trigger substantial financial penalties if this course continued. A nurse-led interprofessional team designed and implemented a Heart Failure Transitions Pilot around a core of evidence-based nurse care coordination interventions. The pilot successfully reduced readmissions to 9% estimated at a cost savings during the pilot year.

As the first new program designed to prepare the Carondelet system for new payment incentives and penalties, it was essential that the project team identify and share key steps in program development and implementation. This would set the stage for scaling up care coordination programs, including successful application for Carondelet to participate in a national value-based purchasing initiative. Each of the following four steps was seen as integral to the success of the Heart Failure Transitions Project: Step 1. Create consensus on the care delivery model; Step 2. Operationalize key processes in the model; Step 3. Build a set of preferred post-acute and community providers who partner in model implementation; and Step 4. Incorporate effective and efficient use of technology.

Step 1. Creating Consensus on the Care Delivery Model

One of the first steps in creating the model for the Heart Failure Transitions Project was to identify major stakeholders and experts in transitional care for this population. The initial project team consisted of leadership and staff from Carondelet's community health programs, medical staff, and cardiology groups. Carondelet's vice president for Community Health and Continuum Care, a nurse with extensive leadership in case management and administration, was designated as team leader. Several cardiologists who were members of Carondelet's practice agreements with local cardiology groups agreed to serve as advisors for the project. Carondelet's chief medical officer was pivotal in engaging primary care physicians and specialists in the program design and execution.

The Carondelet Heart Failure Advisory Committee convened with three primary objectives: 1) to develop the community-based model for the pilot; 2) to define the tools and the protocols; and 3) to provide oversight of the implementation and evaluation plan. The final Advisory Committee consisted of four cardiologists, the chief medical officer for the Carondelet Medical Group, the Health Information Management director, and the hospital network's chief medical officer, with the vice president for Community Health and Continuum Care serving as committee organizer and facilitator.

The Advisory Committee reviewed a number of models that included a nurse practitioner-led outpatient clinic and a more community-based approach such as the Transitional Care Model (Naylor, 2004) which utilizes advanced practice nurses in a community setting to manage high-risk patients over a 60-day period post-discharge. Key elements in the Transitional Care Model include:

- A focus on patient and family engagement and building their level of confidence in their care
- Patient and family education and self-management training
- Medication reconciliation and management
- Monitoring and support that continues from hospital to post-acute settings (Naylor, 2004)

Transitional Care Nurses and the Navigator

Over the course of several meetings, the team decided that a modified Transitional Care Model would be the preferred community model that the cardiologists would support. The model was modified to utilize cardiology nurses as transitional care nurses (TCNs) rather than nurse practitioners. These nurses were considered nurse experts based on their years of experience and advanced professional education in nursing leadership. In the modified model, the TCNs worked with a community health outreach worker called the navigator. The navigator role was envisioned as a non-professional person who was well-regarded in the community and would provide care coordination support for the nurse.

Step 2. Operationalizing the Model

The major interventions in the Heart Failure Transitions Project were those delivered by the transitional care nurse and navigator who bridged between hospital care and post-acute care. They work closely with hospital staff, primary care providers, specialists, and community services. The TCNs and the navigator used a standardized assessment and intervention model, called the FAST approach to organize their interventions (FAST is explained on page 192).

The TCN is the heart of the program providing clinical expertise and care coordination leadership (See sidebar on page 193: A Day in the Life of a Transitional Care Nurse). This role includes self-management education, medication reconciliation, and care coordination for heart failure patients in their community setting for up to 60 days. The TCN visits patients in their homes, skilled nursing facilities, and assisted living homes and work in tandem with home health nurses when patients were receiving home care. The TCNs attend cardiology appointments with patients post-discharge offering coaching at the visit and serving as a "second ear" for the patient.

The TCNs provide patients in the project with telehome monitoring scales for daily monitoring of weight. These scales have Bluetooth capability to transmit the patient's weight to a cellular device located in their home. This device then transmits the weight to a website that health professionals can access with a password for HIPAA protection. Patients in the project are asked to keep daily logs in which they record their heart failure symptoms. The logs include ratings of symptoms within green, yellow, and red zones that reinforce progress and alert patients and families when a call to a primary care provider or specialist is indicated. The navigator also assists the patients with appointment making, data tracking, and telehome monitoring.

The TCNS and navigator also play an important part in the design and continuous improvement of the Heart Failure Program. The TCNs and the Advisory Committee were engaged from the beginning in tool development and program evaluation. It was important that the tools capture and measure key processes of care, as well as the intended quality and cost outcomes. The TCNs and Advisory Committee researched a number of assessment tools including those intended to capture risk for rehospitalization and patient confidence in caring for themselves. They reviewed available tools to monitor patient self-care activities and activate actions, such as contacting a primary care provider or cardiologist with weight gain. Most commonly, standardized measures were used for outcomes, like hospital readmission rates. All of the tools also were examined for their use in web-based documentation for the project.

The project team chose to include a patient risk assessment tool, a patient rating of self-care confidence based on Lorig's (2013) self-efficacy measure, and a chronic illness knowledge survey. The risk assessment tool was used to match the intensity of patient intervention to their likelihood of being rehospitalized. Individuals who scored higher on the risk tool were scheduled for home visits as well as telephonic visits. The self-care and knowledge tools provided important information about the patient's knowledge of symptoms, diet, medications, and help-seeking to guide patient-centered interventions. Monitoring tools were modeled from Wagner's (2006–2013) Chronic Care Model that uses a stoplight framework for alerts. The team incorporated standardized outcome tools, including the CDC Quality of Life Questionnaire (CDC, 2011), the New York Heart Association (NYHA) Guidelines for Staging of Heart Failure (NYHA 1994), and satisfaction surveys for patients and physicians routinely used within the Carondelet system.

FAST Approach to Disease Management

The heart failure team utilized the FAST approach (Lamb & Zazworsky, 2000) for their disease management methodology. The acronym FAST stands for: Find; Assess; Stratify; Treat, Train, and Track.

- *Find:* The nurses utilized various means to find patients. This included in-patient referrals from physicians, case managers, and staff nurses, as well as computer-generated lists for diuretics and readmissions within the last six months.

- *Assess:* The nurses utilized a risk assessment tool that incorporated evidence-based measures related to the NYHA guidelines for heart failure, the patient's self-rating of their health, reported co-morbidities, and laboratory parameters.

- *Stratify:* The nurses stratified patients into low, moderate, and high risk groups deploying a risk appropriate intervention grid (see Table 1).

- *Treat, train, track:* The nurses led the efforts in developing the heart failure log and zone tools with the Heart Failure Advisory Committee physicians. Patients were taught these tools while they were still in the hospital and during their home visits with the TCN. The TCN also administered a level of confidence tool to guide self-management education. The patients also

The Day in the Life of a Transitional Care Nurse
by Amy Salgado, MS, RN

After being a charge nurse on the cardiac floor for many years, I was ready for a challenge. Working as a transitional care nurse was a real eye opener the first year. As a floor nurse you did not get the full picture on how the patient functioned and what the challenges were in their home environment. Patients were often classified as noncompliant when seen in the hospital. Being able to go into the patient's home, it became clear that what we were calling noncompliant was far more complicated. The social issues out in the communities were huge. Many times we had to hold off on patient education until we addressed some of the social issues, such as food, medications, housing, family dynamics, and transportation, that created significant obstacles for patients caring for themselves or being able to adhere to self-care guidelines. Providing meaningful and useful education was also a huge challenge. Patients were given a pre- and post- confidence and knowledge test to determine what areas of self-management needed work. The pre-test tools were administered as soon as the patient left the hospital. Our pre-and post-test measurements showed that there was a lot of education needed for the patients and their families. Many patients left the hospitals not sure about their disease process, medications, diet, and strategies to stay out of the hospital.

Being a transitional care nurse has been very rewarding and fulfilling. Learning to work with different cultural and learning styles of patients, families and physicians has been quite an adventure. Many times there was resistance with the primary interactions from both patients and physicians. Once everyone started to understand that we were experienced and knowledgeable, our relationships with these individuals became very encouraging and interactive. Many patients enjoyed the relationship with a knowledgeable and experienced professional and did not want to leave the program. The physicians noticed the difference in their patients particularly when the nurse came to the physician visit with the patient. The patients were prepared with their logs and questions—creating a more proactive and engaged visit. As a result, the physicians started referring more patients to the program.

received a colorful patient education booklet on heart failure. The goal was to keep it simple for the patient. All materials are at the fourth- to fifth-grade level, culturally appropriate, and available in English and Spanish. Recognizing that many of the patients were Hispanic, it was important that a TCN and the navigator were also bilingual in Spanish.

Table 1 Risk Intervention Grid in Carondolet's FAST Approach to Disease Management

Low Risk	Moderate	High
HF Daily Log and Zones	HF Daily Log and Zones	HF Daily Log and Zones
Telephonic calls by our team (transitional care nurse, social worker, and navigator)	Telephonic calls by our team (transitional care nurse, social worker, and navigator)	Telephonic calls by our team (transitional care nurse, social worker, and navigator)
Coordination of services: ■ Primary and specialty visits ■ Social needs	Coordination of services: ■ Medical nutrition therapy ■ Primary and specialty visits ■ IV intervention at outpatient infusion therapy ■ In-home social needs	Coordination of services: ■ Medical nutrition therapy ■ Primary and specialty visits ■ IV intervention at outpatient infusion therapy ■ In-home social needs
	Medical nutrition therapy	Medical nutrition therapy
		Telehome/Web-based monitoring of weight, blood glucose, O_2 saturation, and blood pressure
Chronic Disease Navigation Portal (web-based tracking)	Chronic Disease Navigation Portal (web-based tracking)	Chronic Disease Navigation Portal (web-based tracking)

Strategies also were designed to encourage continued physician engagement in the project. Many of these tactics relied on timely and effective communication by the TCN with physicians during hospitalization and through the transitional care period. Evidence-based tools were developed to support clear and consistent communication about the plan of care and patient follow-up activities.

Step 3. Building Preferred Providers across the Continuum

Parallel to the implementation of the Carondelet Transitional Heart Failure Program, a post-hospital strategy was created to facilitate transitions of care through preferred provider arrangements with key skilled nurse facilities, home health, and infusion therapy partners. These continuum partners with aligned values and quality services were invited to participate in our pilot preferred provider process. Each partner was asked to enter into an agreement that would promote transitions of care and quality. These preferred providers were also placed on Carondelet's preferred provider list that is given to hospitalized patients along with the list of all post-hospital providers when post-hospital care is ordered.

Currently, Carondelet's preferred providers participate in bimonthly meetings and report quality and readmission data. In addition, the preferred providers utilize Carondelet's patient education materials and transition protocols.

In early 2012, the local Area Agency on Aging's Pima Council on Aging (PCOA) approached Carondelet to partner on a care transitions program that they were recently awarded, based on the Care Transitions Intervention (CTI) model developed by Eric Coleman. This model includes several key features about patients during care transitions:

■ *Medication self-management:* The patient is knowledgeable about his/her medications and has a medication management system.

■ *Use of a dynamic patient-centered record:* The patient understands and utilizes the personal health record (PHR) to facilitate communication and ensure a continuity of care plan across providers and settings. The patient or informal caregiver manages the PHR.

■ *Primary care and specialist follow-up*: Patient schedules and completes follow-up visits with the primary care physician or specialist physician and is empowered to be an active participant in these interactions.

■ *Knowledge of red flags:* The patient is knowledgeable about indications that their condition is worsening and how to respond." (Parry, Coleman, et al., 2003)

Recognizing the need for more community-based support, Carondelet entered into an agreement with the PCOA to provide health coaching with many of the heart failure patients post-discharge. PCOA offers an array of social and community case management services that will augment the clinical components of the care transitions work and offer extended services after the care transitions period.

Step 4. Using Technology

Telehome monitoring was a crucial addition to the transitional care program. Many times the patient would be asked what their current weight was and the TCN would be told "You know… the same… 140." The TCN would then make a home visit and see that the patient was very edematous and short of breath. Obviously, the patient had not been weighing himself. The telehome scales helped provide the accountability to help the patient understand when they were going into heart failure. The nurses would help reinforce the heart failure zone and support the patient in their self-management. This provided a real-time component to the program. TCNs and navigators are able to log into the telehome monitoring web site on a daily basis and see the patients' weight or see if they have not weighed themselves. Telehome blood pressures and pulse oximeters are also part of the program to assist with the patients that have been diagnosed with acute myocardial infarction (AMI) and pneumonia.

Another technology component that was developed was the Chronic Disease Navigation Portal. This is a web-based documentation tool for the TCNs, social workers, and navigators. The team can now chart as they are out in the patients' homes. This helps the team see what has been done, what is still needed, and report the findings on their visits. This also provides an immediate look at what the team is doing and the challenges that they may be facing in the patients' homes. The plans are to have this portal integrate with the hospital-system's Electronic Health Record in the near future.

MOVING INTO A CMS COMMUNITY-BASED CARE TRANSITIONS PROGRAM

In April 2011, the Center for Medicare and Medicaid Services (CMS) announced funding for acute care hospitals with high readmission rates that partner with community-based organizations (CBOs) that provide care transition services to improve a patient's hospital-to-home transition. Section 3026 of the Affordable Care Act, the Community-based Care Transitions Program (CCTP) was established to test models in order to improve care transitions from the hospital to other settings for high-risk Medicare beneficiaries. This program would use CBOs, such as the local Area Agencies on Aging, to partner with hospitals to provide the community-based intervention to manage care transitions

With Carondelet experiencing success in their initial efforts and having already partnered with the local Area Agency on Aging, both entities decided to pursue the CMS opportunity. The reason to expand was apparent. Carondelet needed to increase their footprint in reaching the number of Medicare beneficiaries who were at-risk for readmissions and make a greater impact on their high Medicare 30-day readmission rates. This opportunity would allow Carondelet to expand their efforts and help transform their care transitions efforts for value-based purchasing.

In March 2012, Carondelet was selected by CMS to become one of their Community-Based Care Transitions Program across the country. Their partnership with PCOA serving as the community-based organization offered a strong network of social and outreach services. As a result, this new program manages patients with a broader range of chronic illnesses including heart failure, AMI, pneumonia, COPD, diabetes, renal, and skilled nursing facility (SNF). Although SNF discharges are not a disease, a root cause analysis demonstrated that patients discharged to a SNF had an increased rate of readmissions within the first 7 to 14 days post-discharge. Therefore, it was decided that SNF discharges would be included in the expanded program discharges.

Called the Carondelet–Pima Council on Aging Transitional Care Navigation Program, or Care Transitions Program, this new effort expanded the initial efforts of

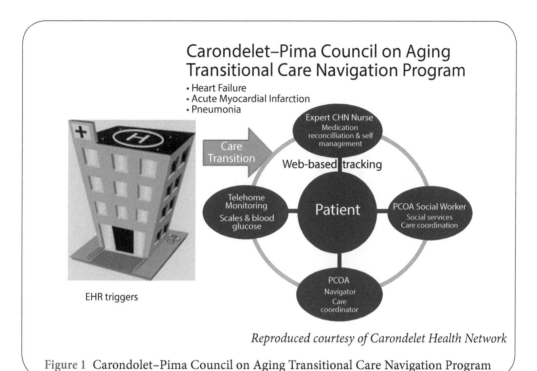

Figure 1 Carondolet–Pima Council on Aging Transitional Care Navigation Program

the Heart Failure Care Transitions Program, building on the coordinated system of care with a community-wide effort (see Figure 1). The Care Transitions Program incorporates many of the features tested in the Heart Failure Project, including risk assessment for readmission, evidence-based patient education tools, telehome monitoring scales, and transitional nurses and navigators to provide self-management support, medication reconciliation, and care coordination during the care transitions.

New elements were added to the program to round out a system-wide effort that starts at the time of admission and extends through the discharge and care transitions period. These new elements include:

- A multidisciplinary community-based team of nurse experts, social workers (called health coaches), and community health outreach workers called navigators (see Figure 1).

- Expansion of the technology to include the web-based portal called the Chronic Disease Navigation Portal and telehome monitoring devices to include scales, blood pressure cuffs, and oximeters. The Portal allows the community-based team to document their interventions in real-time, enabling the team to know the various clinical and social interventions underway for the patient. The web-based tools allow the nurses to enhance

self-management capabilities to include pneumonia, COPD, renal, and
AMI.

■ A community coalition that includes Carondelet, Pima Council and
Aging, preferred providers (skilled nursing facilities, home health, and
infusion therapy), community agencies (mobile meals, behavioral health
agencies), and the University of Arizona Center on Aging. The coalition
meets quarterly to review the progress of the Care Transitions Program in
reducing readmissions.

■ The ReEngineering Discharge Process or RED (Jack & Brickmore, 2010–
2011) for the hospital's discharge process. This is a 12-step process that
defines the roles and responsibilities of the hospital team to accomplish a
successful discharge. These steps include defining who reviews the medications with the patient prior to discharge, who does "teach-back" with
the patient on their disease and self-management needs, who reviews the
patient's test results and follow-up needs, and, finally, who makes the follow-up appointment with the physician (primary care or specialist) seven
days post-discharge.

■ A "Virtual Ward" to track care transitions patients post-discharge for 60
days while they are in the program. The virtual ward is embedded in the
EHR. Also, by having these patients in the virtual ward, the ED providers
are triggered with a "red flag" if a care transitions patient comes into the
ED during these 60 days post-discharge.

■ An expansion of diagnoses to include heart failure, acute myocardial
infarction, pneumonia, COPD, renal, and SNF referrals.

■ The expectation of performing root cause analysis to determine causes for
all readmissions. The community-based team and preferred providers are
expected to complete a root cause analysis on any readmission. This has
allowed the team to perform rapid cycle improvements such as targeting
social interventions more appropriately in high-risk social situations.

LESSONS LEARNED

Implementing community-based care transitions programs requires nurses to consider
a number of issues in clinical and program management. Nurses are key facilitators in
program development, implementation, and improvement, as well as the hub for the

delivery of patient care. As nurses embrace these challenges, there are some lessons learned in this journey.

- *Provide structure, but allow for flexibility.* In the first year, the nurses, along with the Advisory Team, established a practice framework, but found that as the program evolved, many new realities needed to be addressed. For example, the nurses were spending half of their time on social issues in order to help patients with their medical conditions, so it was critical to build a social worker component into the program. During the second year, the team had to evolve their model in order to increase the volume of patients served. This involved restructuring the risk assessment and intervention grid to distinguish between high medical versus high social risk. Now the transitional care nurse who screens the patients in the hospital assesses risk and assigns patients to different providers according to their immediate needs. The transitional care nurse visits patients who are high-risk in their medical and health issues, while the social worker visits patients who are high-risk in their social needs. The team may do a joint visit if the patient is high-risk for both medical and social issues. All others receive a telephonic intervention, unless the nurse or social worker determines that a home visit is necessary.

- *Provide time for team building with community partners.* It is a natural phenomenon for a team to experience bumps along the way. Therefore, it is important for the team to have time to process together in a safe environment that respects the various disciplines that are needed to carry out care transitions work. It is important for the nurse to provide a leadership role in not only establishing regular sessions for processing, but also providing the group structure in which to process. This includes helping the team to identify and prioritize the issues and allowing the team to guide the solutions.

- *Educate, educate, educate.* Develop a five-minute elevator talk. The TCN provides on-going education to staff nurses, physicians, and community agencies. It is never ending. New staff and physicians need to be oriented to the program immediately—on the spot, particularly on how to make appropriate referrals. Our community agencies, such as skilled nursing facilities' staff need to be educated on when to contact the transitional care nurse or social worker to help prevent a hospital readmission. They also need on-going education on the patient education tools and how to utilize them appropriately. It is a never-ending process; therefore, the nurse must become proficient in describing and encouraging the use of the program quickly and clearly.

- *Lead the change.* Providing care transitions is a work in progress. Therefore, establishing rapid cycle improvement processes is critical to the success of any program, but particularly with care transitions work. The TCN leads this change through on-going root cause analysis for every readmission. The TCN must provide this leadership in order to change individual and system processes that could be at the root of the problem. For example, heart failure patients were being readmitted to the hospital because of fluid overload. As the transitional care nurse became involved, it was identified that home intervention with IV diuretics could avoid an emergency room visit. So the TCN worked with the physicians to provide this intervention. The TCN also identified a home infusion company that could perform the home visit within four hours of the order. Now, hospitalizations are avoided with this new service.

CONCLUSION

On a local level, with a year experience as a CCTP funded program, Carondelet and PCOA have demonstrated positive results in both reducing readmissions of the Medicare population served and expanding the program footprint with the addition of more diagnoses. This community-based partnership has been a learning laboratory not only blending care transitions models but also building team cohesiveness and role clarification. The nurse's role will continue to evolve in care coordination and program leadership as the model evolves. The balance of managing more patients in their community setting requires continuous quality improvement in their structure and processes.

On a national level, as these programs continue to take shape, hospitals will experience the positive aims that the Affordable Care Act set out to achieve—improved quality while reducing costs. Nurses are equipped to provide the team leadership needed in both the hospital and community settings.

As these programs continue to move from the demonstration context to an established program within the healthcare system or community, there are several issues to consider. Can these programs be scaled at the local level? How will they continue to be funded? What role will the nurse play in these models? Answers to these questions depend on the flow of funding through cost avoidance or plan contracts in order to sustain these programs. In any circumstance, nurses must maintain a seat at the table and be the voice for the patients.

REFERENCES

Centers for Disease Control and Prevention (CDC). (2011). Control quality of life questionnaire. Retrieved from http://www.cdc.gov/hrqol/hrqol14_measure.htm#1

Jack, B., & Bickmore, T. (2010–2011). The re-engineered hospital discharge program to decrease rehospitalization. *Care Management*, 12–15. Retrieved from http://www.bu.edu/fammed/projectred/publications/CMdec2010jan2011.pdf

Lamb, G., & Zazworsky, D. (2000). Improving outcomes FAST. *ADVANCE for Post-Acute Care*, 3(1) 28–29.

Lamb, G., & Zazworsky, D. (2005): The Carondelet story. In E. Cohen and T. Cesta (Eds.), *Nurse case management* (3rd ed.) (pp. 581–590). Maryland Heights, MO: Mosby.

Lorig, K. (2013). Chronic disease self-management program. Retrieved from http://patienteducation.stanford.edu/programs/cdsmp.html

Naylor, M. D., Brooten, D. A., Campell, R. L., Maislin, G., McCauley, K. M., & Schwartz, J. S. (2004). Transitional care of older adults hospitalized with congestive heart failure: A randomized controlled trial. *Journal of the American Geriatrics Society*; 52, 675–684.

New York Heart Association (NYHA). (1994). Guidelines for heart failure: The criteria committee of the New York Heart Association. In *Nomenclature and criteria for diagnosis of diseases of the heart and great vessels* (9th ed.) (253–256). Boston, MA: Little, Brown, & Co.

Parry, C., Coleman, E. A., Smith, J. D., Frank, J. C., & Kramer, A.M. (2003). The care transitions intervention: A patient-centered approach to facilitating effective transfers between sites of geriatric care. *Home Health Services Quarterly, 22*(3), 118.

Wagner, E. (2006–2013). Improving chronic illness care. Group Health Research Institute. Retrieved from www.improvingchroniccare.org

ACKNOWLEDGMENTS

A special thanks to Donald Denmark, MD, Sr. Vice President, and Chief Medical Officer, Carondelet Health Network; Amy Salgado, RN, MS, Transitional Care Clinical Coordinator; Jim Murphy, PCOA CEO, and the Carondelet-PCOA teams for their vision, expertise and commitment for the success of our program.

Chapter 12

Influencing Public Policy through Care Coordination Research

Marilyn Rantz, PhD, RN, FAAN; Lori Popejoy, PhD, RN;
Katy Musterman, MBA, RN; and Steven J. Miller, MA

As people age, they want to live at home—not in nursing homes or assisted living facilities—retain as much independence and health as possible (Marek & Rantz, 2000; Rantz, Marek, Aud, Johnson, et al., 2005a; Rantz, Marek, & Zwygart-Stauffacher, 2000). In an effort to keep older adults at home for as long as possible, family members will often provide needed services, including care coordination. In 2009, the cost of caregiving by family members in the United States had an estimated value of $450 billion (AARP, 2013a). Giving care to older adult family members is challenging. Most family members are not trained to coordinate care, navigate the healthcare system, nor are they knowledgeable about how to best help older people maintain or regain health and independence. Furthermore, many family members do not live close to their older adult relative, making it challenging to monitor their condition and coordinate care from a distance (AARP, 2013b). When family members are not able to care for their loved ones, older adults often find themselves living in traditional long-term care facilities.

Traditional models of long-term care that include nursing homes and assisted living facilities are not uniformly accepted by older adults and their family members. The baby boom population is rapidly aging and is demanding new models of care that maximize independence and optimize physical functioning to enable better quality of life for community dwelling older adults. As with every other social institution in the U.S., the baby boomers have also shifted the vision of long-term care: they are demanding ways to age successfully without moving to a nursing home. The University of Missouri (MU) Sinclair School of Nursing (SSON) stepped up to the challenge of creating a different way of supporting older adults as they age, providing care on their own terms. Working with stakeholders, including consumers, politicians, community leaders, and long-term care advocates, MUSSON opened a home healthcare agency and partnered with Americare Systems, Inc. to build a new senior living community focused on care coordination. This new model of care is called Aging in Place (AIP) and implementation of the model required strategic planning for shifting public policy, ongoing project effectiveness evaluations, stakeholder involvement, building a business for the AIP project, developing the care coordination program, passing legislation to enable building a demonstration site, building and operating the demonstration site, and overcoming challenges to diffusion of the care model. The goal of AIP is to allow older people to remain in the environment of their choice for as long as they wish without fear of forced relocation to a higher level of care (assisted living or nursing home) (Marek & Rantz, 2000; Marek, Rantz, & Porter, 2004).This chapter will discuss how public policy was successfully influenced by engaging others to create a much-needed new model of care coordination for older adults living in the United States.

KEY STEPPING STONES TO ULTIMATELY INFLUENCING PUBLIC POLICY

The Vision: Dramatically Change U.S. Long-Term Care Delivery

Although the AIP project began with a clearly stated vision from the outset, there were many stepping stones to success. The primary goal of the project, envisioned by MUSSON in 1996, was to change public policy in order to transform how long-term care is delivered in the United States. At that time, there were two major public policies that inhibited development of new solutions to better meeting the long-term care needs of older adults: 1) Regulations that force institutional care into categorical service "boxes" such as senior housing, residential care, group homes, assisted living, intermediate care, nursing facilities, skilled nursing, long-term acute care, acute rehabilitation, etc.; and 2) Regulations that limit payment for RN or APRN care coordination in home and community-based or facility-based long-term care.

An interdisciplinary group was selected and convened to guide the project. An initial ground-rule was to *not* let current public policies inhibit envisioning a new model of long-term care for older people. The group identified the typical path for older adults as transitioning from home to assisted living then to nursing homes as their health and functional abilities decline. It was recognized that once an older adult moves to a long-term care setting (assisted living or nursing home), state and federal regulations determine the amount and type of services that must be provided: if a person requires more care than allowed under the regulations, the person is forced to move to a higher level of care (Marek & Rantz, 2000; Rantz et al., 2000). For example, in assisted living, a person must be able to navigate a path to safety without assistance or he or she is required to move to a higher level of care. Research shows that each move is detrimental to the person's well-being, often resulting in reduced functioning (Manion & Rantz, 1995). Older adults who move to assisted living facilities or nursing homes rarely return to living independently in the community. The only exception to this is when older adults are admitted for a short stay in a nursing home for rehabilitation, such as what would be needed after a fall with a hip fracture (Bentler et al., 2009). Once permanent admission to higher levels of care begins, the trajectory is a slippery slope resulting in the loss of independence and the need for more institutionalized care (see Figure 1).

The new model envisioned by MUSSON faculty allowed an older person to *age in place*, staying in the environment of their choice with key services *coming to them* as they age *via nurse care coordination*. The foundation was carefully built on the nurse care coordination research of the community nursing organizations that used the model of nurse care coordination, nursing home diversion demonstration projects of the 1970s and early 1980s, and the Robert Wood Johnson Teaching Nursing Home Initiative of the late 1980s.

To actually operationalize the model, it was necessary to gain a better understanding of what others thought was possible, to better understand the limitations of current public policy regulations, and to determine possible alternatives that included changing regulations. Toward that end, MUSSON faculty made site visits to innovative housing and community-based models of care in other states that were considered best practice long-term care sites, meeting with providers from a variety of disciplines and backgrounds. Additionally, long-term care advocates, geriatric researchers, community leaders, and consumers were instrumental in defining the AIP model. The resulting model included

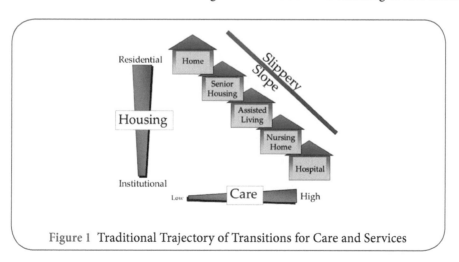

Figure 1 Traditional Trajectory of Transitions for Care and Services

best practice community-based health care with intensive registered nurse (RN) care coordination (Rantz et al., 2011). The vision also included the construction of elder housing for implementation of the AIP model within an ideally constructed environment (TigerPlace, named after the MU mascot) where people could age in place without being forced to move to higher levels of care as their needs increased.

Building a Business for the AIP Project: Sinclair Home Care

After three years of business and research planning, MUSSON received a $2 million grant from the Centers for Medicare and Medicaid Service (CMS) to establish a home care agency and evaluate the AIP model of care. As a result, in 1999, Sinclair Home Care, a Medicare and Medicaid certified home health agency was established as a department within MUSSON.

The key service provided in AIP is RN care coordination, a service not paid for at that time by Medicare or Medicaid. The CMS grant provided funding for this service for Medicare, Medicaid, and private pay clients of the home care agency so that the AIP model of RN care coordination could be evaluated for cost and clinical outcomes. The RN care coordinator manages the client's care needs across time, disciplines, and services (primary care, specialty care, social work, physical therapy, hospice, and others) regardless of payer, enabling the client to age in place. The mission statement of Sinclair Home Care reflects the dedication to the ideal of keeping older adults in the community home of their choice and states that the agency will promote the independence, dignity, and health of adults by providing the services and support needed for them to live in the home of choice. Sinclair Home Care is dedicated to the enhancement of the quality of life of clients served through the delivery of compassionate health care by skilled professionals continuously striving for excellence.

For 10 years, Sinclair Home Care provided Medicare and Medicaid home health services to six counties in the mid-Missouri region using nursing care coordination. Additionally, private pay services were available in one county. Services included skilled nursing care, medication management, wound care, nurse on-call services, personal care services, and physical, occupational, and speech therapies. RN care coordinators communicated with clients' physicians, therapists, and other caregivers to ensure that care was appropriate and necessary. As with many home healthcare agencies during this period, after the CMS-funded community-based AIP research was complete, it was challenging for Sinclair Home Care to remain profitable while continuing to provide what we knew was important to better care, the now "unfunded" care coordination work. Since it was no longer necessary, for evaluation purposes, to continue to operate a home health and home- and community-based services business, on July 1, 2009, the Medicare and Medicaid components of Sinclair Home Care were sold to Oxford Healthcare by MU Health Care. MUSSON retained the private pay business which continues to provide AIP care coordination and home care services to TigerPlace residents; this facilitates ongoing evaluation of AIP at TigerPlace, as well as research activities and educational programs.

Strategic Planning for Shifting Public Policy: Electronic Health and Business Databases

With a clear vision to influence public policy, several implementation stepping stones were essential:

- Use an electronic health record for periodic data analysis of care delivery that included standardized data elements that enabled comparisons with traditional long-term care;

- Plan all data collection so it is doable, useful, and occurs within the normal workflow of the nursing staff and other employees;

- Use periodic comparison groups in the community and with state and national databases; and

- Publish ongoing results of evaluations that are of interest to policy makers because topics such as cost, quality, and staffing are addressed.

Project Effectiveness Evaluations: Building the Case to Influence Public Policy

It was necessary to obtain effectiveness data about AIP that would later be used to influence legislators. The outcomes of the CMS evaluation (1999–2003) demonstrated that clients who received care from Sinclair Home Care with RN care coordination had improved clinical outcomes compared with individuals of similar case-mix in nursing homes (Marek et al., 2005). Outcomes were also significantly better for clients with RN care coordination than without RN care coordination in a community-based waiver program called Missouri Care Options (MCO) (Marek, Popejoy, Petroski, & Rantz, 2006). Monthly costs to Medicare were significantly lower ($686) for MCO clients with RN care coordination compare to those without care coordination (Marek, Adams, Stetzer, Popejoy, & Rantz , 2010). Finally, total costs to Medicare and Medicaid were $1,592 lower per month in the AIP group than a nursing home comparison group over a 12-month period (Marek, Stetzer, Adams, Popejoy, & Rantz, 2012). These documented cost savings and better clinical outcomes proved useful as efforts to change public policy progressed.

Challenging Existing Paradigms: Legislation to Enable Building TigerPlace

Clearly, the outcomes of AIP in the community were positive; now the challenge was to leverage the research outcomes to enable changes in Missouri long-term care regulations so TigerPlace could be built and operated in a new paradigm. The AIP vision always included having an ideal housing environment where older adults could live and receive excellent care and services. It was extremely challenging to build a new kind of facility that offered increased resident autonomy, service, and care coordination within the highly regulated long-term care industry. It became apparent that if the vision of a building was to become a reality, new regulations had to be written. Based on the positive initial results of the CMS AIP evaluation, legislation was proposed and passed in 1999 and 2001 which established four demonstration sites for AIP in Missouri. MUSSON and Americare Systems, Inc. applied for and became one of the demonstration sites and TigerPlace is the only remaining AIP demonstration site.

Involving Stakeholders: The Public-Private Partnership

Passage of the legislation and actual implementation of the public policy change required engaging all stakeholders. Before the legislation was proposed, an attempt was made to involve any person with an interest in the proposed legislation. This included those interested in preserving the status quo.

Marilyn Rantz, PhD, RN, FAAN, a faculty member at MUSSON, took the lead in the AIP project and began meeting with key stakeholders. Tim Harlan, a state representative, took an interest in the project and Dr. Rantz met with Mr. Harlan and officials of the Missouri Department of Health and Senior Services to draft potential legislation for a demonstration project. After months of meetings and ongoing communication through email and phone calls, drafts were ready for discussion. Dr. Rantz discussed the potential legislation with other crucial stakeholders, including the representatives from the nursing home associations (Missouri Health Care Association and Missouri Association of Homes and Services for the Aged), the ombudsmen, the Area Agency on Aging, and other state legislators.

Mr. Harlan began meeting with his legislative colleagues to build support for the law. In addition, advocates who were also stakeholders began calling legislators endorsing the law. It was essential that consensus about the proposed change be established before bringing the legislation to the floor for a vote. While some associations were hesitant to endorse the new law, they did agree to not oppose the legislation, which was critical in its passage. Through the combined efforts of all of the interested parties, the legislation that enabled the AIP program finally passed in 1999 and 2001. After passage of the law, MUSSON continued to work with state officials and in partnership with Americare Systems, Inc. to build TigerPlace as an AIP demonstration site.

The public–private partnership between MU and Americare is unique. In order for the partnership to work, the two entities needed a shared vision and an understanding of the care model and the role each would fulfill. Through considerable discussion, legal agreements were established to delineate the roles and responsibilities of each party. This ongoing relationship building continues to the present with representatives from MUSSON and Americare meeting monthly to discuss operational issues.

Building the Demonstration Site: TigerPlace as AIP Long-Term Care Facility

In 2004, construction was completed for TigerPlace. Designed as an ideal environment for AIP, it is operated by Americare with home care services provided by Sinclair Home Care. To enable people to remain in the same apartment as they age and as care needs change, it was decided to license TigerPlace as an Intermediate Care Facility (ICF), thus enabling residents to use their long-term care insurance when they qualify. The building was built to nursing home standards (with some waivers that enable the environment to not appear "institutional") with private studio, one-, and two-bedroom apartments and is operated as an independent living community. Americare provides housekeeping, maintenance, two meals per day, and transportation services. Sinclair Home Care provides RN care coordination including: an RN on call 24 hours a day; comprehensive healthcare assessment on admission, every six months, and as needed when physical or mental health significantly changes; medication management; wellness checks; personal care services; and health promotion activities including exercise classes at TigerPlace. Unlike typical ICF care, there are legal exceptions in place for the license that allows residents to receive care and services at TigerPlace as their needs change, without requiring them to move to a higher level of care. Residents of TigerPlace can stay there through the end-of-life, so they can truly age in place (see Figure 2).

Domestic pets have been an integral part of TigerPlace since the beginning. The planning team recognized the important benefits of pets for older adults and TigerPlace residents are encouraged to have them (Johnson, Rantz, McKenney, & Cline, 2008). There is a veterinary clinic on site, which is staffed by the MU College of Veterinary Medicine.

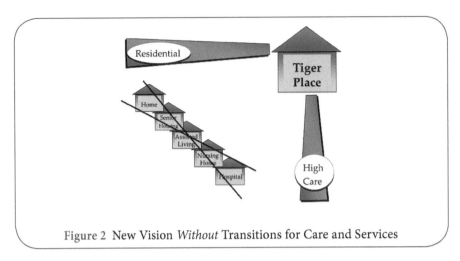

Figure 2 New Vision *Without* Transitions for Care and Services

Veterinary and nursing students assist residents in caring for their pets by walking dogs, administrating medications, and feeding animals whose owners are in the hospital or receiving rehabilitation in other facilities. A veterinarian does monthly rounds to check on resident pets and offer advice to residents with issues or concerns. The residents rest easy knowing that their pets will always be taken care of if they become incapacitated or after they die because there is an adoption policy in place at TigerPlace.

Care Coordination:
Central to Sinclair Home Care Services at TigerPlace

The care service line provided at TigerPlace is a home healthcare RN care coordination model combined with routine client assessments that effectively catch problems early so that interventions to restore optimal health can be provided. A wellness center is open five days per week and is available to all residents of TigerPlace. Services provided at the wellness center include vital sign checks, assistance with minor health problems, and registered nurse consultation for residents and families. The majority of care takes place in the resident's apartment. Residents pay privately for home care services such as medication management, assistance with activities of daily living, personal care services such as bathing and dressing, and wound care. Residents are assessed upon admission, every six months, and as needed based on physical and mental health needs. If residents meet Missouri's ICF criteria, they are evaluated more frequently and receive an increased amount of RN care coordination to maximize their independence and health.

Sinclair Home Care arranges for services to restore and maintain optimal health. When residents are ill or have periods of lower functioning, they receive increased services, which are removed when residents are able to return to their higher level of functioning. This reduces overall care costs and encourages clients to maintain or improve their health and functional ability. RN care coordination is provided to all residents as a part of the overall wellness package. The RN care coordinator works with residents' care providers and family members to address potential and actual health concerns. The goal is to communicate potential problems so that interventions can be put into place before they lead to acute illnesses and hospitalizations.

The direct care pricing models changed when AIP moved from the community to a congregate housing setting. Instead of hour-long home health aide or nurse visits, visits were priced in smaller increments so an aide (or nurse) could complete tasks over several "visits" in the apartment throughout the day or week. This worked for a few years, then the pricing model was changed to a package structure to better support frequent short visits, improve use of staff time, and accommodate for individualized care in the AIP model. As a result of transitioning to a package structure, client satisfaction improved because the costs to the client were more predictable. The AIP services at TigerPlace through Sinclair Home Care are a stable and viable business operated by MUSSON.

Social work services have been an integral part of AIP since the inception of Sinclair Home Care. A licensed clinical social worker (LCSW) is available to help with counseling, community resource linkages, and other forms of psychosocial support. The LCSW assists with mental health and psychosocial assessments, advance directive planning, client social histories, and provides support with hospice care. The LCSW and RN care coordinator maintain a close working relationship when care planning with residents and their families. The integration of nursing and social work has maximized communication and an ability to view the residents in a holistic way that promotes early interventions.

More Project Effectiveness Evaluations: AIP at TigerPlace

A subsequent evaluation of the first four years of the AIP program at TigerPlace and another senior housing community receiving AIP services from Sinclair Home Care revealed significant cost savings and health improvements over traditional long-term care (Rantz et al., 2011). The combined care and housing cost for any resident who received care services beyond AIP basic services (routine assessment, access to the wellness center, exercise classes, and other health promotion activities) and who qualified for nursing home care has never approached, nor exceeded, the cost of nursing home care at either location. Subsequent evaluations have found that both mental and physical health outcome measures provide evidence that AIP is an effective model for health restoration and independence for older adults through the end-of-life.

Technological Innovations: Technology to Enhance AIP

As the construction of TigerPlace was being planned, a challenge was posed to the engineering faculty at MU by Dr. Rantz for them to work with nursing and other faculty to develop new solutions to the persistent problems facing older adults. Specifically, they were challenged to develop technology that would help older adults stay as healthy and functionally independent as possible.

Working with older adults, the research team developed unobtrusive sensor technology that would monitor individuals as they performed every day actions (Rantz et al., 2005b). The participants do not wear any devices or perform any specific actions. The resulting integrated sensor network includes motion sensors, video sensors including the Microsoft Kinect, and a bed sensor that captures pulse, respiration, and restlessness as the resident sleeps. A web-based interface was developed to display the data from the sensors in a way that is easy to use, easy to understand and interpret, and clinically relevant (Alexander et al., 2011). Integrated sensor networks have been installed in over 50 apartments at TigerPlace. See Figure 3 for a diagram of this network.

The goal of the sensor network was to support care coordination at TigerPlace. The interdisciplinary Eldertech research team has accomplished this goal and more (Rantz et al., 2010; Rantz et al., 2012). The technology developed and implemented by the Eldertech team detects changes in function and health status of older adults and alerts staff to those changes so proactive interventions can manage healthcare problems in early stages, when interventions are most effective.

Using the sensor data, clinicians detect early changes in health conditions including urinary tract infections, increased congestive heart failure, changes in mental status, and many others before traditional healthcare assessment (Rantz et al., 2012). Based on the clinicians' observations and a retrospective analysis, alerts generated from the sensor data were developed with input from the nursing and engineering faculty. A one-year, two-group pilot study (people living with sensors and those living without) was completed using the sensor network to detect changes in health status indicating an impending acute illness or exacerbation of a chronic illness. In that pilot study, the care coordinator and other clinicians received these alerts; when warranted, the nurse or LCSW would assess the resident and intervene as necessary. Intervention participants living with the sensor networks showed significant improvements as compared to the control group in the Short Physical Performance Battery gait speed score at quarter 3 ($p=0.03$), average left hand grip at quarter 2 ($p=0.02$), average right hand grip at quarter 4 ($p=0.05$), and the GAITRite (a sensor mat that analyzes participants' gait while simply walking on it) functional ambulation profile at quarter 2 ($p=0.05$) (Rantz et al., 2012).

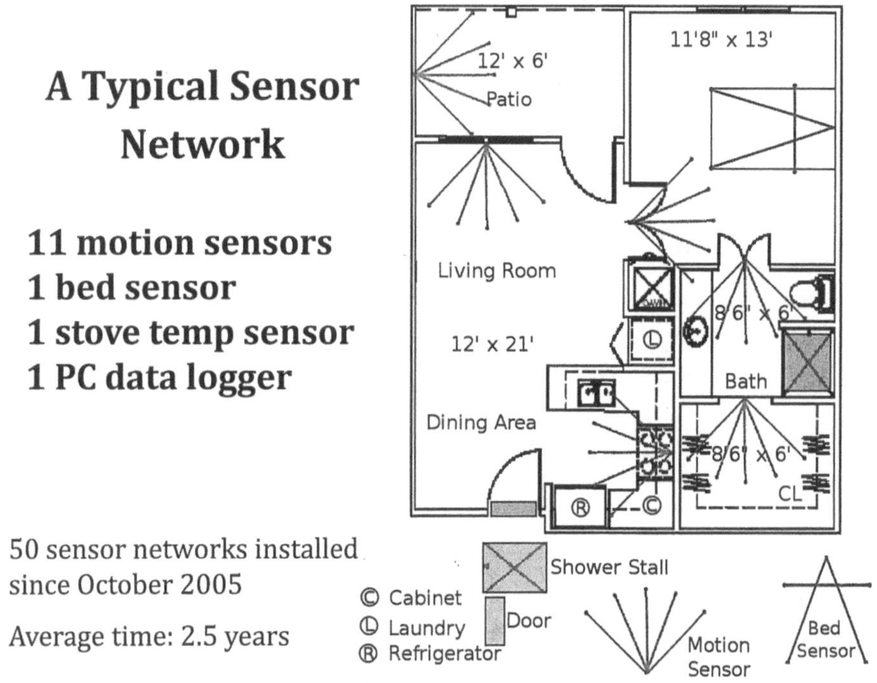

A Typical Sensor Network

11 motion sensors
1 bed sensor
1 stove temp sensor
1 PC data logger

50 sensor networks installed since October 2005

Average time: 2.5 years

Reproduced with permission of Sinclair Home Care Aging in Place

Figure 3 Integrated Sensor Networks at TigerPlace

Based on the results of the pilot study, the integrated sensor network has been incorporated into the usual care at TigerPlace. The sensor technology is used as a decision support system for care coordination; it augments traditional healthcare assessment by facilitating earlier detection of illness and exacerbation of a chronic illness. It is now being tested in a large scale clinical trial funded by the National Institute of Nursing Research and the technology is now being commercialized so others can benefit from the technological innovations.

Challenges to Diffusing the Care Model: Becoming a National Long-Term Care Model

Based on the success of TigerPlace, Americare Systems, Inc. is planning another AIP facility in the Missouri region and working with MUSSON as planning progresses. This is the first step to widespread adoption of AIP throughout the country. Many other organizations and companies have been onsite to discuss the model at TigerPlace for replication in their locations. They have learned about TigerPlace through national publicity of the research about AIP, as well as the extensive technological innovations research.

The operations team at TigerPlace has willingly offered their expertise and assistance to others to replicate or innovate the RN care coordination model. When people visit, they clearly state that TigerPlace is a national model for a new long-term care environment.

There were many challenges for AIP to overcome to receive this recognition. Foundational are the care coordination cost, quality, and staffing evaluations about AIP in the community and at TigerPlace. Those evaluations have drawn attention to the effectiveness and cost savings of RN care coordination as an effective care delivery model regardless of setting. In addition to the challenges of operations and evaluations, the main challenge was business viability for the community-based services.

In the original 1999–2003 evaluation funded by CMS, the RN care coordination model was developed and used in public housing, private homes, and congregate housing. The grant supported the RN care coordination costs and the typical care was funded by the Medicaid Home and Community Based Services. After the grant concluded, to help the agency be viable as a business, more profitable services such as private pay and private insurances balanced the challenges of limited Medicaid funding. Even with that business approach, it was extremely challenging for the home care agency to break even on costs using public reimbursement mechanisms such as Medicaid and still provide the much needed care coordination.

Today, it is likely that recent Medicare funding approval for care coordination will improve the business viability of the RN care coordination using the AIP model in public housing. Specifically, there are now mechanisms to bill for "complex chronic care coordination services." These "services are patient-centered management and support services provided by physicians, other qualified healthcare professionals, and clinical staff to an individual who resides at home or in a domiciliary, rest home, or assisted living facility… the reporting individual provides or oversees the management and/or coordination of services, as needed, for all medical conditions, psychosocial needs, and activities of daily living" (AMA, 2013, p.35). This would considerably reduce the challenges faced ten years ago to constantly seek grant funding or donations to support the critically important RN care coordination function for the elderly and disabled. With new deployment today in public housing situations, it is likely some modifications to the model will have to be made to best fit current reimbursement policies.

The Cutting-Edge Challenge:
Staying Alive Until Change Becomes Widespread

As a cutting-edge program, there are no others out in front to watch, learn from, and anticipate challenges to be expected in the future. The operations team has to work closely and constantly keep the goal of helping older adults maintain independence through the end-of-life in focus in all clinical situations. It can be easy to revert to traditional solutions for older adults who are experiencing health changes or events that may pose safety hazards. These traditional solutions are often encouraged by primary care providers and usually involve moving to a higher level of care such as assisted living or nursing homes. There is a belief that traditional long-term care will somehow solve safety problems like falling.

Constant education about the AIP model of care that encourages independence and health promotion is needed to remind other healthcare providers, families, residents, surveyors, and sometimes our own team members that residents living at TigerPlace can be independent while also receiving safety and care measures thought only to be available in traditional care facilities. Staff members working in the AIP model make extraordinary efforts to promote resident independence, decision-making, and maintenance of maximum physical and cognitive function through the end-of-life.

However, because the care model is cutting edge, consumers, healthcare providers, and regulators not familiar with AIP try to "make it fit" into some traditional "box" or typical category of traditional assisted living, nursing home, or housing concept. Surveyors not experienced in evaluating TigerPlace and the approach to care often struggle to understand it. When surveyors conduct the annual inspection, they are often confused because traditional care systems are replaced by care coordination, health promotion activities, and independent decision-making by residents. It is a lively, dynamic model of care delivery that looks very different from the usual facilities that surveyors visit. Until the AIP care model with RN care coordination is more widespread, explanation and education will be a constant part of daily operations.

What to Do When You Are the Only One

It is essential that organizations providing new and unique models of care continue to work with stakeholders (lawmakers, physicians, visiting scholars, nurses, families, and the clients served). *Keep involving stakeholders* to reinforce and renew the vision and involve the next generation of leaders (undergraduate and graduate nursing students, engineers, social workers, informaticians, new healthcare providers, and others) so they can continue, distribute, and improve upon the model.

Focus on innovation. The constant focus on innovation promotes an openness to new ideas so the care services can improve and be more efficient and effective. The focus on innovation in AIP have resulted in building an electronic health record that supports care coordination by improving documentation of care delivery, communication, and functional status. Simultaneously, this electronic healthcare record serves as a continuous source of data to support research and evaluation. A major innovation has been the development of sensor technology to enhance the wellbeing and functional status of older adults.

Continuously promote the project through personal communication, publications, and presentations. Take the time to develop fresh summary documents (flyers, pamphlets, short news articles) about the services, outcomes, and innovations developed by the new model of care. While it takes time to tour people through the organization, that time is critical to promote and spread the word from person to person. Talk to colleagues, policymakers, and others, leaving summary briefs for them to remember the project at a later time. Publish the results in journal articles and press releases. Present results at local, national, and international conferences. Talk to community stakeholders and groups. Open the doors to the organization so that visitors can see the model and envision a new way of thinking about care delivery.

Know When to Change

Nothing remains static. Health care is dynamic and the forces that shape healthcare delivery are under constant pressure to change. It is critical to keep abreast of changes on the state and national horizon and be positioned to respond to changes. When pressures appear to be potential problems for operating the innovative care delivery model, stop and decide: (a) Must something be done? (b) If so, what? and (c) How aggressive should the response be? The model will need to evolve and ultimately the day may come when a decision for radical change must be made. If that happens, work with an operations team to guide the project as a business and as an evolving innovation. Teams make better decisions than single decision makers, especially in cutting edge innovations.

SUCCESSFULLY INFLUENCING PUBLIC POLICY

The TigerPlace AIP experience has illustrated four key steps toward successfully influencing public policy.

Take Expert Advice Seriously.

About three years ago, AIP team members were urged to prepare short videos of the RN care coordination and costs results of the AIP innovations and cost-effectiveness evaluations. These were not easy to plan and do, but three different versions were produced and captured the ideas well enough for ANA and the American Academy of Nursing (AAN) to use as they pursued influencing CMS to change policies about Medicare funding for care coordination. It is rewarding to know that the efforts of the AIP evaluation and communicating the results effectively in the three-minute videos had at least some part in getting Medicare regulations changed for RN care coordination for those with complex chronic care needs. Care coordination was specifically addressed in one section of the Medicare regulations (AMA, 2013, p. 35) and there is opportunity for a second change in the transitional care management services:

> These services are for an established patient whose medical and/or psychosocial problems require moderate to high complexity medical decision-making during transitions of care from an inpatient hospital setting (including acute hospital, rehabilitation hospital, long-term acute care hospital, or skilled nursing facility/nursing facility, to a patient's community setting (home domiciliary, rest home, or assisted living). (AMA, 2013, p. 36)

With these funding mechanisms, there is potential for the RN care coordination innovation to help millions of other older adults.

Publicize the Results

MU has consistently distributed both written and video press releases which have been syndicated by news outlets, television and radio, and professional publications throughout the country. Scholarly articles about the evidence of cost, quality, and outcomes of RN care coordination and technology innovations at TigerPlace were written to publicize the results in peer-reviewed journals. In addition, an AAN Edge Runner application was prepared. Using the ongoing evaluation results, the AIP Project and TigerPlace received an Edge Runner designation in 2008. The application materials have been updated to keep them current for use for public policy briefs.

Continuously Engage Stakeholders

Stakeholders must be consistently updated about the progress of the innovative care delivery models so they can maintain enthusiasm for the innovations. Routinely engage them in conversation and share important information about the program. For TigerPlace, an AIP Advisory Board was established at the beginning of the project in 1996 and the group of about 20 diverse community stakeholders continues to meet quarterly. The Board is made up of community aging advocates, Missouri Department of Health and Senior Services representatives, faculty and staff of the University, and others. Board members help build and maintain positive relationships with the community at large to help provide continuous community recognition and support for the TigerPlace innovations. Communication and relationships are critical to project success.

It is essential that lawmakers who are key stakeholders stay engaged. The AIP Board is chaired by the legislator (now retired) who sponsored the aging in place legislation in 1999. As a former legislator, he helps explain the project and build continued support for it with current legislators. He helps keep local, state, and national representatives informed about the original intent of the legislation backing the project and the positive contributions the project has made to health care. Results about cost savings and improved outcomes for older people are of interest to legislators. The operations team at TigerPlace also engages current legislators in conversations and they often tour the site; they get to know staff and residents personally and appreciate the positive results of the innovation. The team and board members take every opportunity to explain the work and showcase the service.

From the outset, national nursing organizations (American Academy of Nursing, American Nurses Association) and CMS were involved. Ideas were shared early and often. Results about outcomes of care and costs were shared as they were measured, articles written, and press releases circulated.

Most importantly, the voices of clients need to be heard. Satisfaction surveys are helpful, but frequent private interviews with residents and families can provide much needed insight to their needs and desires. The AIP and TigerPlace central goal is to keep older adults happy and healthy, promoting the highest quality of life as idealized by the individual; this is impossible to do without their input.

Always Engage in Public Policy Change

Although there are now Medicare mechanisms to fund care coordination, there are still remaining issues that need to be addressed through public policy change. The primary issue at this stage is to enable and facilitate the construction of long-term care facilities that continuously promote health, regaining independence when functional decline occurs, and enable older people to remain in the one place to receive care services as their needs change. There are state-specific hurdles for spreading the success of AIP at TigerPlace by replicating the building and care delivery model across the country. In Missouri, with regulatory waivers and state statute changes, the construction and evaluation of AIP at TigerPlace was enabled over 10 years ago. Now, it is time for other states to replicate it so that consumers have access to this cost- and clinically-effective new model of long-term care. Some states are well-positioned with long term regulations and state regulators who are interested in pursuing a different approach. Other states will require changes in building and operational regulations to enable construction of this independent living environment that enables getting the right services at the right time through the end-of-life, without fear of unwanted relocation.

CONCLUSION

The key to moving demonstration projects into public policy is the rule of the 3Ps: Persistence, Persistence, and Persistence. The process is long and arduous. It takes hours of meetings, presentations, and conversations. But in the end, the work is necessary and worthwhile especially when it improves the lives of older adults and their families.

REFERENCES

AARP. (2013a). Valuing the invaluable: 2011 Update. The growing contributions and costs of family caregiving. Retrieved from http://assets.aarp.org/rgcenter/ppi/ltc/i51-caregiving.pdf

AARP. (2013b). Providing care: Obstacles to long-distance caregiving. Retrieved from http://www.aarp.org/relationships/caregiving-resource-center/info-09-2010/pc_obstacles_to_long_distance_caregiving.html

Alexander, G. L., Wakefield, B. J., Rantz, M., Skubic, M., Aud, M., Erdelez, S., & Al Ghenaimi, S. (2011). Passive sensor technology interface to assess elder activity in independent living. *Nursing Research,60*(5), 318–325. PMCID: PMC3272505.

American Medical Association (AMA). (2013). CPT Codes for evaluation and management. See http://www.ama-assn.org/ama/pub/physician-resources/solutions-managing-your-practice/coding-billing-insurance/cpt.page

Bentler, S. E., Liu, L., Obrizan, M., Cook, E. A., Wright, K. B., Geweke, E. A...Wolinsky, F. D. (2009). The aftermath of hip fracture: Discharge placement, functional status change, and mortality. *American Journal of Epidemiology, 170*, 1290–1299. doi: 10.1093/aje/kwp266

Johnson, R. A., Rantz, M. J., McKenney, C. A., & Cline, K. M. C. (2008). TigerPlace: Training veterinarians about animal companionship for the elderly. *Journal of Veterinary Medical Education, 35*(4), 511–513. PMID: 19228901.

Manion, P. S., & Rantz, M. J. (1995). Relocation stress syndrome: A comprehensive plan for long-term care admissions. *Geriatric Nursing, 16*(3), 108–112.

Marek, K. D., Adams, S. J., Stetzer, F., Popejoy, L., Petroski, G. F., & Rantz, M. (2010). The relationship of community-based nurse care coordination to costs in the Medicare and Medicaid programs. *Research in Nursing & Health, 33*, 235–242. PMCID: PMC3046776.

Marek, K., Popejoy, L., Petroski, G., Mehr, D., Rantz, M. J., & Lin, W. (2005). Clinical outcomes of aging in place. *Nursing Research, 54*(3), 202–211.

Marek, K. D., Popejoy, L., Petroski, G., & Rantz, M. J. (2006). Nurse care coordination in community-based long-term care. *Journal of Nursing Scholarship, 38*(1), 80–86.

Marek, K., & Rantz, M. J. (2000). Aging in place: A new model for long-term care. *Nursing Administration Quarterly, 24*(3), 1–11.

Marek, K. D., Rantz, M. J., & Porter, R. T. (2004). Senior care: Making a difference in long-term care of older adults. *Journal of Nursing Education, 43*(2): 81–83.

Marek, K. D., Stetzer, F., Adams, S. J., Popejoy, L., & Rantz, M. (2012). Aging in place versus nursing home care: Comparison of costs to Medicare and Medicaid. *Research in Gerontological Nursing, 5*(2), 123–129. PMID: 21846081.

Rantz, M. J., Marek, K. D., Aud, M. A., Johnson, R. A., Otto, D., & Porter, R. (2005a). TigerPlace: A new future for older adults. *Journal of Nursing Care Quality, 20*(1), 1–4.

Rantz, M. J., Marek, K. D., Aud, M. A., Tyrer, H. W., Skubic, M., Demiris, G., & Hussam, A. A. (2005b). A technology and nursing collaboration to help older adults age in place. *Nursing Outlook, 53*(1), 40–45.

Rantz, M. J., Marek, K. D., & Zwygart-Stauffacher, M. (2000). The future of long-term care for the chronically ill. *Nursing Administration Quarterly, 25*(1), 51–58.

Rantz, M. J., Phillips, L., Aud, M., Marek, K. D., Hicks, L. L., Zaniletti, I., & Miller, S. J. (2011). Evaluation of aging in place model with home care services and registered nurse care coordination in senior housing. *Nursing Outlook, 59*(1), 37–46. PMID: 21256361.

Rantz, M. J., Skubic, M., Alexander, G., Aud, M., Wakefield, B., Koopman, R., & Miller, S. (2010). Improving nurse care coordination with technology. *Computers, Informatics, Nursing, 28*(6), 325–332. PMID: 20978402.

Rantz, M. J., Skubic, M., Koopman, R. J., Alexander, G., Phillips, L., Musterman, K. I., Back, J. R, … Miller, S. J. (2012). Automated technology to speed recognition of signs of illness in older adults. *Journal of Gerontological Nursing, 38*(4), 18–23. PMCID: PMC3366277.

Author Profiles

Gerri Lamb, PhD, RN, FAAN
Associate Professor, Arizona State University, College of Nursing and Health
Innovation; Herberger Institute for Design and the Arts, Phoenix, Arizona

Recent care coordination highlights:

- Co-chair, National Quality Forum Care Coordination Measures Review Committees, 2008–2009, 2011–2012
- PI: Nurse Sensitive Measurement of Hospital Care Coordination, Robert Wood Johnson Foundation Interprofessional Nursing Quality Research Initiative (INQRI) 2006–2008.
- Director, Community Nursing Organization Demonstration, Funded by the Health Care Financing Administration to evaluate nurse care coordination in a capitated payment model, 1994–1999.

In my years of practicing, studying, and leading care coordination programs, I have come to view care coordination as the hallmark of patient-centered and effective health care. It represents how well our health care system works—or doesn't work—for patients and their families. I am excited and energized to see care coordination recognized as a priority for health reform: this is the impetus nurses and colleagues across health care have needed to propel this important work forward.

CHAPTER CONTRIBUTORS

Corrine Abraham, DNP, RN
Nurse Fellow, VA Quality Scholars Program, Atlanta VA Medical Center; Clinical
Assistant Professor, Nell Hodgson Woodruff School of Nursing, Emory University,
Atlanta, Georgia

Recent care coordination highlights:

- Leading an interdisciplinary team to develop a falls prevention program to minimize modifiable risks for injury across the Atlanta VA Medical Center health system.
- Partnering with interprofessional colleagues to improve the safety and quality of care for veterans afflicted with chronic non-cancer pain managed

with opioid therapy, addressing policy changes, new practice guidelines, data collection/tracking, and new models of care.

■ Serving as coach and mentor for medical residents, nursing residents, and practicing primary care providers in learning QI methods through implementation of quality projects.

My current focus: enhancing local capacity for leading change to achieve improved patient outcomes. In working with several national collaboratives as communities of practice and learning on fall prevention and chronic pain management, I've been able to network with national experts, local leaders, and key stakeholders. My future goal is to bridge the gap between academia and practice by promoting translation of evidence to enhance healthcare delivery and improve patient outcomes, whatever the focus.

Richard C. Antonelli, MD, MS
Medical Director of Integrated Care and Physician Relations and Outreach, Boston Children's Hospital; Faculty, Harvard Medical School, Boston, Massachusetts

Recent care coordination highlights:

■ Consultant on care coordination and integration methodologies and measures to multiple states, U.S. federal agencies, and international stakeholders.

■ Co-authoring, with nursing and social work colleagues, Making Care Coordination a Critical Component of the Pediatric Health System: A Multidisciplinary Framework, supported by The Commonwealth Fund.

■ Currently project funded by the Lucile Packard Foundation for Children's Health to develop a family-reported measure of care integration.

My clinical work has focused on providing comprehensive, family-centered, team-based care for all children, youth, and young adults, but especially for those with special healthcare needs. In this work, I've been impressed that successful care coordination outcomes could be best achieved by creating partnerships with patients, families, and caregivers, and nurtured by interprofessional collaborative relationships with colleagues in nursing, social work, behavioral health, education, and policy.

Gail E. Armstrong, DNP, PhD(c), ACNS-BC, CNE
Associate Professor, University of Colorado College of Nursing, Aurora, Colorado

Recent care coordination highlights:

■ Member of a faculty team teaching interdisciplinary clinical teams from two hospitals in a year-long course in quality, safety and efficiency, including didactic sessions and ongoing improvement work, centered largely on the concepts and logistics of effective care coordination.

■ Integrating quality, safety and concepts of care coordination into pre-licensure nursing curricula.

Care coordination is the heart of cost-effective, high-quality, and safe patient care. Nurses are well positioned to make vital contributions to the important related improvements to quickly evolving healthcare systems.

Patricia S. Button, EdD, RN

Managing Director, Clinical Architecture, The Advisory Board Company, Washington, D.C.

Recent care coordination highlights:

■ National Quality Forum HIT Critical Paths: Care Coordination Technical Expert Panel (2012)

As the healthcare system transitions from a fee-for-service business model to a risk-based, accountable care model, care coordination enabled by technology and evidence-based practices is absolutely essential. The potential for provision of high-quality and cost-effective coordinated care is within our reach!

Karen Jiggins Colorafi, MBA, RN, CPEHR, CPHIT

EHR Nurse Consultant, Healthcare Practice Services, Ltd., Phoenix, Arizona

Recent care coordination highlights:

■ Consultation with ambulatory care practices to select, implement, and optimizeEHRs, allowing them to connect patient needs along the continuum of care with acute care services and community resources.

■ Work with state and national level agencies to ensure congruence with federal guidelines and policies that help Arizona practices make strides towards the national quality agenda.

The intersection of HIT with care coordination is an exciting one. I am encouraged by the innovations in technology that will certainly advance the practice of care coordination. With technology, we can make health care safer and more efficient for clinicians and patients, while offering patient-centered tailoring that far surpasses our current capabilities.

Ingrid M. Hopkins Duva, PhD, RN

Nurse Fellow, National VA Quality Scholars Program, Atlanta, Georgia

Recent care coordination highlights:

- Member, ANA Care Coordination Quality Measures Panel
- Co-PI: Office of Nursing Services RN Nurse Care Manager Diabetes Management Pilot Implementation Project
- PI: Factors Impacting Staff Nurse Care Coordination; a quantitative dissertation research examining structural factors associated with care coordination activities by staff nurses

Since the beginning of my nursing career, through bedside, management and leadership experiences, I have been struck by the perception in nursing that "indirect care activities" may not be as valuable as direct care activities. My work related to care coordination is an attempt to overcome that perception and raise nursing awareness of its critical care coordination rile. I am motivated daily by the national focus on care coordination, a natural platform for nurses to showcase their talents and experience.

Patricia C. Dykes PhD, RN, FAAN, FACMI

Senior Nurse Scientist; Program Director, Center for Patient Safety Research and Practice; Program Director, Center for Nursing Excellence, Brigham and Women's Hospital; Assistant Professor, Harvard Medical School, Boston, Massachusetts

Recent care coordination highlights:

- Recently participated in a multi-site NQF study funded to evaluate the current state of communication of care plans across settings and levels of care.

My passion is using informatics tools to establish links between the work of nurses and positive patient outcomes. For the past two decades, I've focused on building a framework for evidence-based practice and exploring the impact of health information technology on the work of nurses.

Sheila Haas, PhD, RN, FAAN

Professor, Marcella Niehoff School of Nursing, Loyola University, Chicago, Illinois.

Recent care coordination highlights:

- Co-facilitated with Beth Ann Swan and Traci Haynes research to develop dimensions and competencies for care coordination and transition management to be done by registered nurses in ambulatory care (2013).
- Currently, editing with Dr. Swan and Ms. Haynes, the Registered Nurse Care Coordination and Transition Management Competencies Core Curriculum.

- Appointed member of the ANA Care Coordination Quality Measures Panel Steering Committee (2013).

I am convinced that ambulatory care RNs are positioned to do care coordination for complex chronically ill patients. Passage of the Affordable Care Act has provided the incentive to delineate care coordination dimensions and competencies as part of specifying the nursing role and assisting nurses to develop and demonstrate all competencies requisite to the role. Our work with the RN-CCTM role will enhance the quality and continuity of care in ambulatory settings and enhance patient-centered care across all settings.

Rosemary Kennedy, PhD, RN, MBA, FAAN

Associate Professor, Associate Dean of Strategic Initiatives, Thomas Jefferson University, Jefferson School of Nursing, Philadelphia, Pennsylvania

Recent care coordination highlights:

- Chair, National Quality Forum, Critical Paths: Care Coordination project (DHHS-funded) to assess the readiness of electronic data and HIT systems to support care coordination (2012).
- PI, Acute-to-Home Care Nursing Handoffs: Distributed Cognition Across Patterns of Knowledge (2011)

With care coordination being recognized as a priority for national health reform, there is a tremendous opportunity for nurses to use health information technology to provide patient-centered quality care. In addition, through data mining techniques, the positive impact nurses have on care coordination can be measured and quantified leading to creation of a learning healthcare system. I am excited to move this work forward.

Laura Heermann Langford, PhD, RN

Director, Nursing Informatics, HWCIR, Intermountain Healthcare; Assistant Professor (Clinical), College of Nursing, University of Utah Salt Lake City, Utah

Recent care coordination highlights:

- Co-Chair, HL7 Patient Care Working Group, Care Plan Initiative, Care Plan Domain Analysis Model, Coordination of Care Services Specification Project (2010–present)
- Co-Chair, IHE Patient Care Coordination Technical Committee, Patient Care Plan Content Profile (PtCP) (2013)
- Committee Member, S&I Framework, Transitions of Care and Longitudinal Coordination of Care Initiatives (2011–present)

Care coordination is the key to providing health care at the highest quality for the lowest cost. Nurses play a key role in care coordination and can provide an experienced voice on how policy and standards should be written and applied to improve health care. I am excited to see nursing take a lead in changing our future.

Steven J. Miller, MA
Business Manager Sinclair Home Care Aging in Place, University of Missouri, Columbia, Missouri

Recent care coordination highlights:

- Project Manager for the NIH–NINR-funded project, Intelligent Sensor System for Early Illness Alerts in Senior Housing, a randomized clinical trial of technology to enhance care coordination and early illness detection for residents in senior housing and assisted living.

Since 2005, I've been involved with Sinclair Home Care Aging in Place, where we focus on RN care coordination to help older adults age in place by providing home care services as needed and coordinating care across all disciplines. As the Business Manager, while I'm not directly involved in care coordination, I can see its importance in the lives of the clients.

Katy Musterman, MBA, RN
Manager of Nursing Services Aging In Place, TigerPlace Care Coordinator, University of Missouri Columbia, Missouri

Recent care coordination highlights:

- Currently part of the research team for the NIH–NINR-funded, Intelligent Sensor System for Early Illness Alerts in Senior Housing, a randomized clinical trial of technology to enhance care coordination and early illness detection for residents in senior housing and assisted living.

As the TigerPlace RN Care Coordinator and Manager of Nursing Services for Aging in Place since 2010, I enjoy working with older adults on a daily basis to help them maintain active and independent lifestyles. My operationalization of the AIP model, by working with the residents of TigerPlace to keep them in their apartments through the end of life while reducing ER visits and hospitalizations, is especially satisfying.

Lori L. Popejoy, PhD, RN
Associate Professor, University of Missouri, Columbia, Missouri

Recent care coordination highlights:

- PI for NINR-funded study, Care Coordination for Older Adults: Process, Outcomes, and Cost.
- PI for a core proposal, SNF to Home: Re-engineering SNF Discharge funded by AHRQ as part of an R24 grant, Building Patient Centered Outcomes Research: Care Transitions .

■ Co-Investigator for two CMS Innovations studies: Leveraging Information Technology to Guide High Tech High Touch Care; and Initiative to Reduce Avoidable Hospitalizations among Nursing Facility Residents.

I've worked in care coordination research and practice since 1999. In the last 15 years, care coordination has been proven by numerous research studies to improve patient outcomes. Nonetheless, we continue to struggle to reimburse nurses to independently provide care coordination services. My research seeks to identify and describe the detailed day-to-day work activities of nurse care coordinators in order to more accurately quantify, dose, and reimburse for care coordination.

Marilyn Rantz, PhD, RN, FAAN

Curators' Professor, MU Sinclair School of Nursing; Helen E. Nahm Chair, MU Sinclair School of Nursing; University Hospitals and Clinics Professor of Nursing; Executive Director, Aging In Place and TigerPlace; Associate Director, MU Interdisciplinary Center on Aging, University of Missouri, Columbia, Missouri

Recent care coordination highlights:

■ PI for CMS Innovations Initiative, Missouri Quality Initiative for Nursing Homes (MOQI). Key focus: Reducing avoidable hospitalizations of nursing home residents, care transitions, care coordination.

■ PI for NIH–NINR-funded, Intelligent Sensor System for Early Illness Alerts in Senior Housing. Key focus: Randomized clinical trial of technology to enhance care coordination and early illness detection for residents in senior housing and assisted living.

■ Executive Director of Aging in Place, a special project of the Sinclair School of Nursing since 1996. Key focus: RN care coordination for helping older adults age in place in housing of their choice.

I have dedicated my career to improving senior healthcare services, while simultaneously lowering costs. As my research and findings accumulate, I am hopeful for the future. A paradigm shift in how we evaluate people for disease management and health management is underway. This is reflected in our research into environmentally embedded sensor networks: Being able to understand the patterns in people's lives, and to see signs that something is about to happen, then being able to help people before the health event develops and they require extensive treatment, is highly significant to care coordination in these settings.

Gina Rogers

Consultant and Founding Executive Director, Massachusetts Child Health Quality
Coalition (CHQC), Watertown, Massachusetts

Recent care coordination highlights:

- Leading the CHQC Care Coordination Task Force in defining the key elements of and supporting implementation of foundational elements of high-performing pediatric care coordination, and linking them to process, structure, and outcome measures.

- Participating in the Massachusetts Coalition for the Prevention of Medical Errors and Massachusetts Health Quality Partners, both of which involved statewide learning collaboratives that promote patient safety and patient-reported outcomes and experiences at Massachusetts hospitals,

It is the stories I hear from families trying to manage all the moving parts of their wide-ranging "health neighborhoods" that motivates my care coordination work. Their time and dedication to this work, especially those who pass it forward by helping other families and by looking for policy solutions that can help break down the silos that currently exist, are truly inspirational.

Lipika Samal, MD, MPH

Instructor of Medicine, Harvard Medical School; Associate Physician, Division
of General Medicine and Primary Care, Brigham and Women's Hospital, Boston,
Massachusetts

Recent care coordination highlights:

- Investigator on NQF Critical Paths for Creating Data Platforms: Care Coordination Environmental Scan Report

- Panelist, Clinical Documentation to Support Care Coordination, Office of the National Coordinator for Health Information Technology, Department of Health and Human Services, Washington, D.C.

- Panelist, Closed Loop Care Coordination: The Critical Linkages and Shared Concepts, American Medical Informatics Association Annual Symposium, Washington, D.C.

My experience as a primary care physician caring for increasingly older and sicker patients has shown me the importance of care coordination. The lapses in care which I have witnessed during care transitions motivated me to study the problem through health services research. In the future, I hope to develop innovative HIT solutions to overcome barriers to high quality, patient-centered care coordination.

Madeline H. Schmitt, PhD, RN, FAAN

Professor Emerita, University of Rochester School of Nursing, Rochester, New York

Recent care coordination highlights:

- Consultant to Nurse Sensitive Measurement of Hospital Care Coordination, 2006–2008. Robert Wood Johnson Foundation INQRI grant.
- Consultant to Using Research Findings to Improve Nurse Care Coordination Practice and Policy Robert Wood Johnson Foundation. 2009–2010.
- Chair, Expert Panel for Report: Core competencies for interprofessional collaborative practice: Report of an Expert Panel. (2011). Washington, DC: Interprofessional Education Collaborative (AACN, AACP, AACOM, AAMC, ADEA, ASHP).

I view excellent care coordination as a manifestation of effective patient- or community-centered intra-and interprofessional teamwork. My commitment as a scholar and educator over 40 years has been to understand, teach, and work to improve teamwork and team-based care as a means to improving cooperation, coordination, and collaboration in the service of better outcomes. The moral imperative to improve outcomes continues to inspire my efforts.

Cheryl Schraeder, PhD, RN, FAAN

Associate Professor and Director of Policy and Practice Initiatives, Institute for Healthcare Innovation, University of Illinois College of Nursing, Chicago, Illinois

Recent care coordination highlights:

- Member of Steering Committee, National Coalition on Care Coordination (N3C; Social Work Leadership Institute, New York Academy of Medicine).
- Director, Coordinating Center, Medicare Chronic Care Practice Research Network (MCCPRN), CMS planning grant.
- Project Director, Medicare Coordinated Care Demonstration (MCCD), Illinois site, CMS demonstration.

I have long had the vision that primary care for those with chronic illness desperately needs to be improved. I also believe that nurses and physicians working in collaborative teams, using a comprehensive care coordination approach, are most likely to improve such care. Thus, my 25 years spent on collaborative coordinated primary care intervention to improve the health management of chronically ill individuals. For all the research to date, however. we still have much to learn on optimal delivery of such care.

Daryl Sharp, PhD, PMHCNS-BC, NPP

Associate Dean for Faculty Development and Diversity, University of Rochester School of Nursing. Rochester, New York

Recent care coordination highlights:

- Consultant to the Center for Primary Care, University of Rochester Medical Center, Rochester, NY, 2011–present
- Consultant to the New York Care Coordination Program, Rochester, NY, 2008–2013

I am insatiably curious about the influence of nurses' interpersonal skills on patients' experiences of care and their health outcomes. Understanding patients' perspectives requires a tireless commitment to exploring life from their viewpoint, including a willingness to identify gaps in care and a sincere effort to work with the entire health-care team to remedy such gaps. One simply cannot provide person-centered care in the absence of excellent care coordination. This lies at the heart of nursing and is a continual source of vitality and motivation for my work.

Paul Shelton, EdD

Senior Research Specialist, Institute for Healthcare Innovation, University of Illinois College of Nursing. Chicago, Illinois

Recent care coordination highlights:

- Work with a University of Illinois College of Nursing clinical team to assist the State of Illinois Healthcare and Family Services (state Medicaid authority) to conduct quality management and reporting for the CMS demonstration, Money Follows the Person (MFP), the largest Medicaid demonstration of its kind and the next step toward community-based, log-term care programs.
- Staff member, Coordinating Center, Medicare Chronic Care Practice Research Network (MCCPRN), CMS planning grant.
- Senior Research Analyst, Medicare Coordinated Care Demonstration (MCCD), Illinois site, CMS demonstration.

For over 20 years I have had the opportunity to work with teams of clinicians whose foresight and interest to engage in quality efforts have improve the care for their chronically ill patients. Their interest and commitment have enabled me to use and refine my research skills in evaluating outcomes of care provided to chronically ill adults. I am motivated most by the participating patients who have been involved out of their genuine interest in helping others through sharing their stories, their insights about the frustrations and successes of managing their co-morbid illnesses, and their experiences in navigating a fragmented healthcare system that makes it worthwhile.

Nan M. Solomons, MS

Data Analyst, MaineHealth Center for Quality and Safety, Portland, Maine; Doctoral student, Arizona State University College of Nursing and Health Innovation, Phoenix, Arizona

Recent care coordination highlights:

- Dissertation on the influence of social networks on communication and transitional care best practices
- Program evaluator for pilot grant leading to Medicare CCTP grant in which the Area Agency on Aging partnered with Elder Care Services to extend the Coleman model into the community.

Through my dissertation work I have come to realize the efficacy of building relationships among providers across the care continuum to decrease hospital readmission rates. In Maine, these efforts have resulted in fewer hospital readmissions and improved patient outcomes.

Beth Ann Swan, PhD, CRNP, FAAN

Dean and Professor, Jefferson School of Nursing, Thomas Jefferson University, Philadelphia, Pennsylvania

Recent care coordination highlights:

- Co-facilitated with Sheila Haas and Ms. Haynes (2013) research to develop dimensions and competencies for care coordination and transition management to be done by registered nurses in ambulatory care.
- Currently, editing with Dr. Haas and Ms. Haynes, the Registered Nurse Care Coordination and Transition Management Competencies Core Curriculum.
- Author of the November 2012 Health Affairs' Narrative Matters Feature, "A Nurse Learns Firsthand That You May Fend For Yourself After A Hospital Stay."

After my husband suffered a stroke, we were instantly thrown into the "unreal world" of coordinating his incredibly complex care and managing his many transitions. My professional work and personal experience motivates me to advocate passionately for change.

Donna Zazworsky, MS, RN, CCM, FAAN
Vice President, Community Health and Continuum Care, Carondelet Health Network, Tucson, Arizona

Recent care coordination highlights:

- Executive Co-Lead: Carondelet–Pima Council on Aging Transitional Care Navigation Program, A CMS Community-based Care Transitions Program (2012–present)
- Co-Investigator: Diabetes Disease Management Program: An Evaluation of a Health Reform Clinical and Payment Model in Primary Care (2011–present)
- National Speaker on Community Case Management, Care Transitions, Disease Management (1994–present)

As a nurse leader and innovator in community case management, disease management and care transitions for more than 20 years, never before have we seen such an alignment with our healthcare systems, providers and plans around care coordination. This is an exciting time and an important time for nurses to be in the forefront of healthcare transformation.

Index